Performance Nutrition

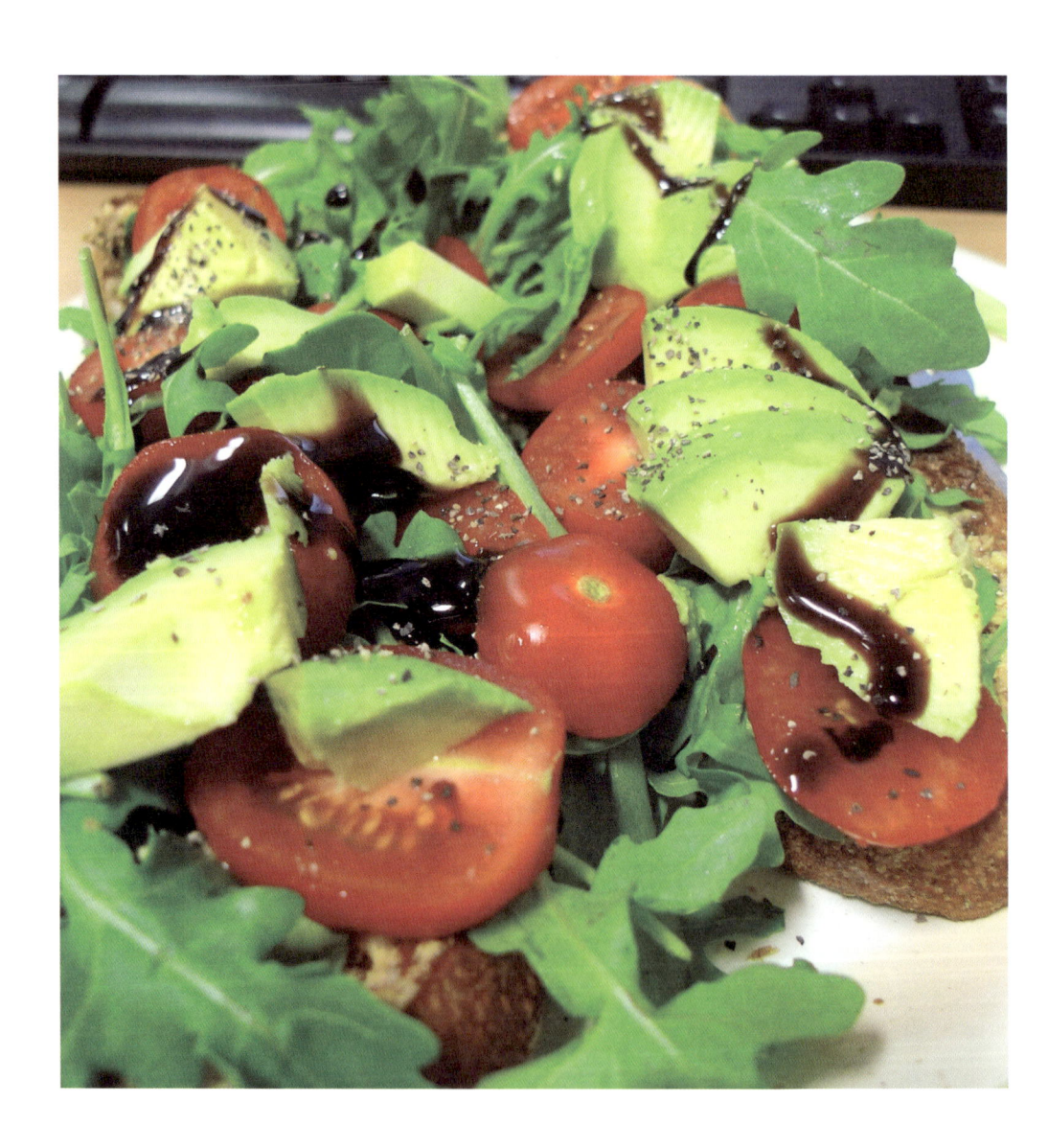

Performance Nutrition

Kevin Currell

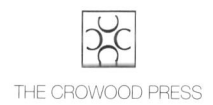

THE CROWOOD PRESS

First published in 2016 by
The Crowood Press Ltd
Ramsbury, Marlborough
Wiltshire SN8 2HR

www.crowood.com

© Kevin Currell 2016

All rights reserved. No part of this publication may be reproduced or transmitted in any form or by any means, electronic or mechanical, including photocopy, recording, or any information storage and retrieval system, without permission in writing from the publishers.

British Library Cataloguing-in-Publication Data
A catalogue record for this book is available from the British Library.

ISBN 978 1 78500 222 9

Frontispiece: Ewan Munro/Wikimedia

Typeset by Jean Cussons Typesetting, Diss, Norfolk

Printed and bound in India by Replika Press Pvt Ltd

CONTENTS

	Introduction	6
1	Preventing Illness	9
2	Nutrition for Injury	22
3	Using Nutrition to Maximize Adaptation to Strength Training	34
4	Concurrent Training and Buffer Capacity	50
5	Maximizing the Adaptations to Endurance Training	60
6	Nutrition and the Brain	76
7	Endurance Events Lasting More Than One Hour	86
8	Events Lasting Less Than One Hour and with Multiple Rounds	106
9	Improving Team Sport Performance	118
10	Weight Management	129
	Index	142

INTRODUCTION

As an athlete, wouldn't it be incredible if you could do something that would give you more time to train, allow the training that you do to be more effective, and enable you to maximize your athletic potential come competition day? Well, there is something that does all of this and more – food.

This book aims to provide an overview of the many areas where food can impact on the performance of an athlete. The approach will be to take an area of performance and explore the role food has.

In Chapters 1 and 2 the focus will be on how what you eat and when you eat influences your health. Chapter 1 will aim to stop you getting ill, while Chapter 2 will try to use food to stop you getting injured. If the worst does happen, it will guide you through how to use food to heal quickly.

Chapters 3, 4 and 5 will explain how to use food to either amplify or dampen the effect of training. Chapter 3 will focus on using food to maximize strength gains, Chapter 4 on how to use food to maximize the effects of concurrent training, and finally Chapter 5 will show you how to use food to obtain gains from endurance training.

Chapters 6 through 9 will focus on pure performance. How food influences the brain and cognitive performance will be the aim of Chapter 6. Chapter 7 will take you through the area of sports nutrition we know most about – endurance performance. Chapter 8 will look at events lasting less than one hour and where recovery is key with multiple rounds. Finally Chapter 9 will look at team sports.

To finish, Chapter 10 will look at weight management in athletes. This is the area where nutrition is commonly regarded as having the most impact, but I hope that reading the preceding nine chapters will have convinced you that food influences much more than just body weight.

Each chapter will start with a tour of the evidence and science on each topic, which makes up the bulk of the text. At the end of each chapter is a simple summary of the potential interventions broken down into the levels of evidence for each intervention, where the categories mean:

- Gold: Very strong evidence from multiple trials showing a positive outcome.
- Silver: Good or emerging evidence that the intervention will influence the outcome.
- Bronze: Weak, but promising evidence that the intervention can influence the outcome.

Following this is an example diet plan for each chapter. If you follow each through you can track the subtle changes that can be made to your diet to influence performance. We will start below with the average intake of our average 70kg male who is not very active. For a female athlete things won't change too much; you are just likely to weigh less so reduce the serving sizes slightly.

INTRODUCTION

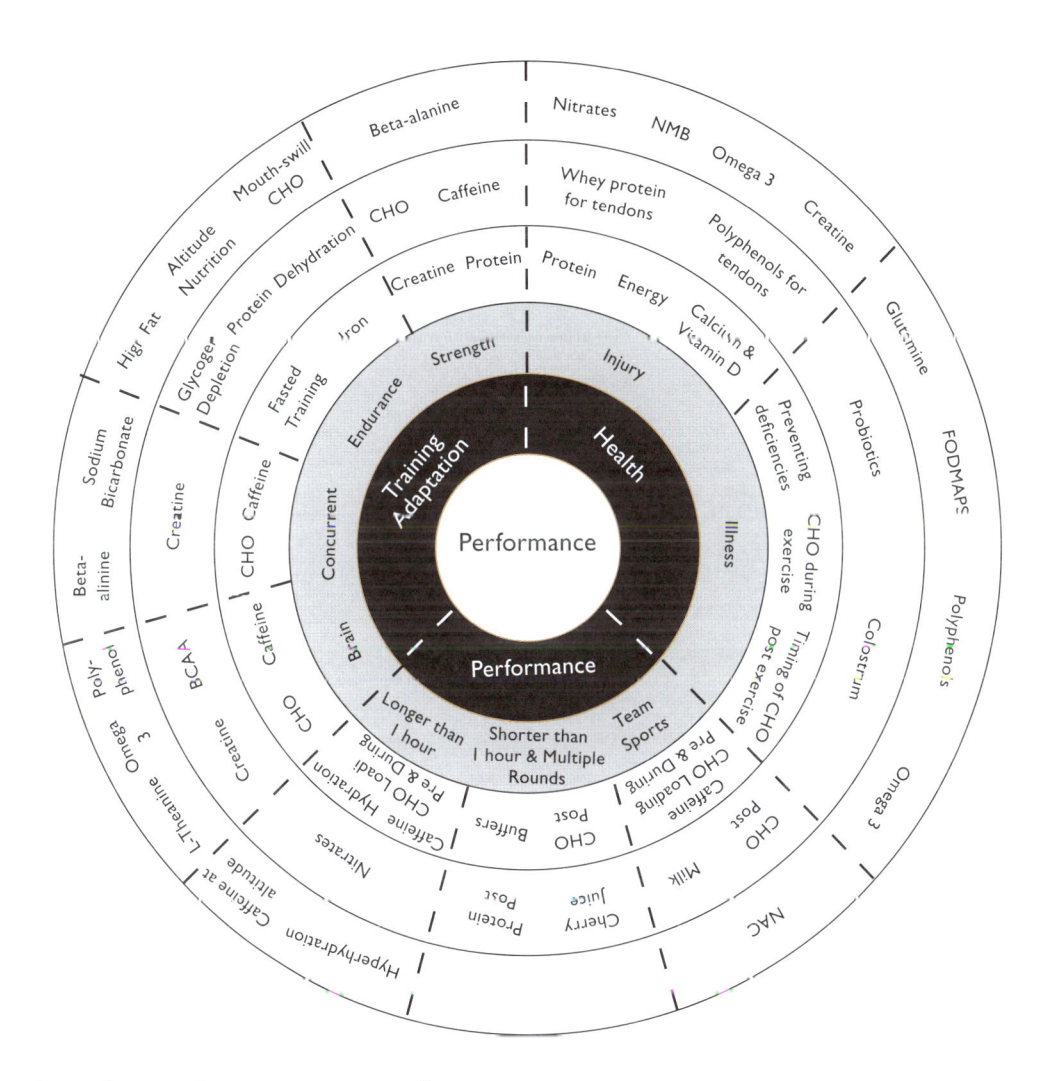

Areas of impact of nutrition on sporting performance.

INTRODUCTION

Meal	Food
Breakfast	Bowl of cornflakes with semi-skimmed milk 1 apple Glass of orange juice Cup of tea with milk
Snack	Packet of crisps and glass of water
Lunch	Egg mayonnaise sandwich on white bread Fruit corner yogurt 1 can of cola
Snack	1 bar of chocolate 1 medium latte
Dinner	Oven-roast chicken breast with oven chips, a green salad with salad cream dressing Ice cream for dessert

Carbohydrate (g/kg body weight) 4.2	Protein (g/kg body weight) 1.2	Fat (g/kg body weight) 1.2

CHAPTER 1

PREVENTING ILLNESS

The barriers were starting to give as the intensity increased. Holes sprung open, allowing easy access for the invading force. Behind the barriers stood the infantry, warriors each of them, waiting, champing at the bit to fight the invading force. Their numbers were increasing as the stress increased and time passed. However, with every passing second and with increasing intensity the defenders were becoming weary, less effective. Behind the infantry, anticipating, prowling, lay the Special Forces – each of them trained to target a particular section of the invading force. Highly trained and specific in what they do, they too were increasing in number, they too were feeling the effects of intensity and time.

No, this is not an action novel. It is a book on performance nutrition. The opening paragraph could also be read as the description of what happens to your immune system when you exercise, whether it is for a long period of time or as intensity increases. Let me introduce you to our characters, the heroes and firstly villains of the story. The invading force is all the bacteria, viruses and parasites that are around us in our day-to-day lives. We never know when we will come into contact with one of these nasties, each of which wants to do us harm. As you read this you are being attacked from all angles. Even the book you are holding will contain some sort of bug that is looking to invade your nice, warm, nutritious body.

Have no fear, though. Your body has developed layers of defence to protect itself from harm. These attacking forces first come up against physical barriers, which must be passed before they can enter the body. These physical barriers include your skin, saliva, nose, stomach and intestine. They are mighty walls of defence. However, each has access pathways and doors through it, otherwise the nutrients you consume in food and the air you breathe would not be able to get into your body. So while there are mighty walls of defence, there are ways through for the invading forces.

When bacteria or viruses or whatever else get past the physical barriers and reach the inside of your body, they come up against a strong, tough infantry, your innate immune system. The infantry will attack all it sees and is not very specific. This infantry is made up of a number of different cells. Neutrophils are the cells that arrive first at a site of infection. Neutrophils use toxic chemicals to neutralize the infection, through a process called degranulation. Macrophages, or 'large eaters' as the original Greek term means, consume and 'eat' invading bugs. Natural killer cells provide protection against your body's own cells, which may have been damaged or taken over by the invading force.

The Special Forces of our immune system form the adaptive immune system. These cells have memory. They remember how best to attack an invader if your body has been attacked before. These are your antibodies, or more technically your lymphocytes.

Exercise acts as a stress on all three parts of

PREVENTING ILLNESS

your immune system, whether it is exercising for a long duration of time or just increasing the intensity of exercise. The physical barriers to infection can become more porous if you exercise for a long period of time. This is best exemplified by the intestine. As you continue to exercise, your intestine becomes more permeable. This increased intestinal permeability allows for easier passage of infection through the intestine. Alongside this there is a decrease in blood flow to the intestine as the blood is redirected to the working muscle. The decrease in blood flow leads to damage being caused to the intestine, further weakening this crucial physical barrier.

Both the innate and acquired immune system follow a similar response to exercise. In particular, after exercise there is first an increase and then a decrease in the number of immune cells available to fight infection. The immune cells that are present, whether infantry or Special Forces, become less effective after exercise.

Athletes do not only train once and then rest. The higher the level, the more they are likely to train multiple times in a day, at high intensities and for long durations. Although at rest there is no difference in the function of the immune system between athletes and non-athletes, there is clearly an effect on the immune system during intensified blocks of training. During these blocks the innate and acquired immune systems can become compromised. In both cases, while there are ample immune cells produced by the body, their function is weakened. This, therefore, increases the risk of infection. Essentially, both the infantry and Special Forces of your immune system cannot function effectively.

A decrease in the effectiveness of the immune system in this way is restored over a period of rest lasting up to two weeks.

On occasion the short-term decrement in immune system function can become a chronic depression. This is a contributing factor to a condition known as overtraining or underperformance syndrome – a long-term period of time where the athlete underperforms for an unknown reason or gets a significant increase in illness.

Exercise is not the only stressor on the ability of the immune army to defend from invasion. What you eat and drink affects the immune system, too. During periods of starvation, or indeed a small energy deprivation, both the innate and acquired immune systems become less effective at fighting infection. Add on top of this dehydration, inadequate protein intake, mineral deficiencies such as copper, iron and zinc, vitamin deficiencies such as vitamins C and E, and the immune system is starting to struggle.

Napoleon Bonaparte once said that 'an army marches on its stomach'. This is true of your immune army, too. It functions on the nutrients with which it is fed; it functions on the energy it is provided with. The food an athlete eats interacts with the training done, and either supports or supresses the immune system. Appropriate nutrition supports the infantry in particular.

Let's start at the beginning, the first line of defence: the intestine. The intestine extends from the stomach to the anus, and is where the vast majority of nutrients and fluids are absorbed. It has two segments, the large intestine and the small intestine. Different nutrients are absorbed at different points along the intestine and by a variety of different mechanisms. However, it is beyond the scope of this book to highlight these many different processes.

The wall of the intestine is made up of four layers. The mucosa: this is primarily the epithelium, which is the innermost wall of the intestine and has direct contact with

PREVENTING ILLNESS

the contents of the intestine. Below this is the sub mucosa, which contains many of the nerves and blood vessels within the intestine. Surrounding the sub mucosa is a layer of smooth muscle, termed the muscularis externa. Finally, comes the serosa, which is the outer wall of the intestine.

The epithelium is where nutrients are absorbed; in the small intestine the epithelium is arranged into a folded pattern, forming villi. This increases the surface area of the intestine, and allows for greater opportunity for nutrients to be absorbed. There are a number of nutrition interventions that can be put in place to help support the intestine during training.

RESEARCH SPOTLIGHT

Energy availability and performance in young female athletes

VanHeest et al. (2014) investigated the effects of ovarian suppression, secondary to an energy deficit, in ten junior elite swimmers (aged fifteen to seventeen). Over a twelve-week period changes were monitored in body composition, energy intake and expenditure, steroid hormones oestrogen and progesterone, metabolic hormones related to thyroid function (total triiodothyronine, TT3), and the metabolic hormone insulin-like growth factor 1 (IGF-1) along with 400m swim time trial performance. The participants were split into two groups: those with menstrual dysfunction and those without. Athletes who had normal menstrual function were in energy balance, whereas those with abnormal menstrual function had on average a 500 kcal per day energy deficit. The outcome of this was a suppression of the hormonal milieu within the body and a decrease in performance over the twelve-week period in the abnormal menstrual group of 9.8 per cent. In contrast, those with a normal menstrual cycle improved their performance over a twelve-week period by 8.2 per cent.

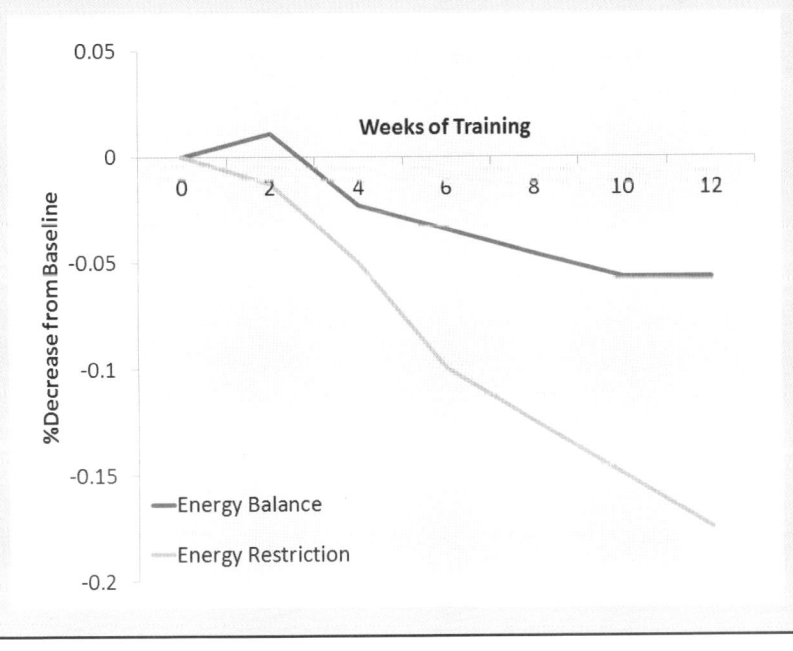

Percentage decrease in total triiodothyronine, TT3, a marker of thyroid function with energy balance or energy restriction over a twelve-week training programme (VanHeest et al., 2014).

PREVENTING ILLNESS

Probiotics

We are not alone. Ever. Our body is populated by over 10,000 different species of bacteria, fungi etc., each playing a role in maintaining various bodily functions. Some of the most well-known reside within the gut, and over the last few years these have been linked to a whole variety of improved health outcomes, including:

- reduced illness
- reduced gastrointestinal illnesses
- reduction in depression
- reduction in inflammation
- helping prevent travellers' diarrhoea
- reduction in colon cancer
- reduction in cholesterol and blood pressure

They sound miraculous, don't they? Now let's not get carried away, because none of these are conclusively proven by any means. What has been interesting, though, are a couple of studies in well-trained athletes, looking at the prevention of illness during heavy training.

The first to really hit the headlines was a paper by Professor Mike Gleeson from Loughborough University. He took eighty-four highly active participants (mainly university students, but there were a few elite athletes chucked into the mix) and split them into two groups. One group drank two Yakult yogurts per day (containing *L.casei* Shirota), every day for four months. The other drank a placebo Yakult, exactly the same in taste and nutrition but not containing probiotics. The results proved interesting.

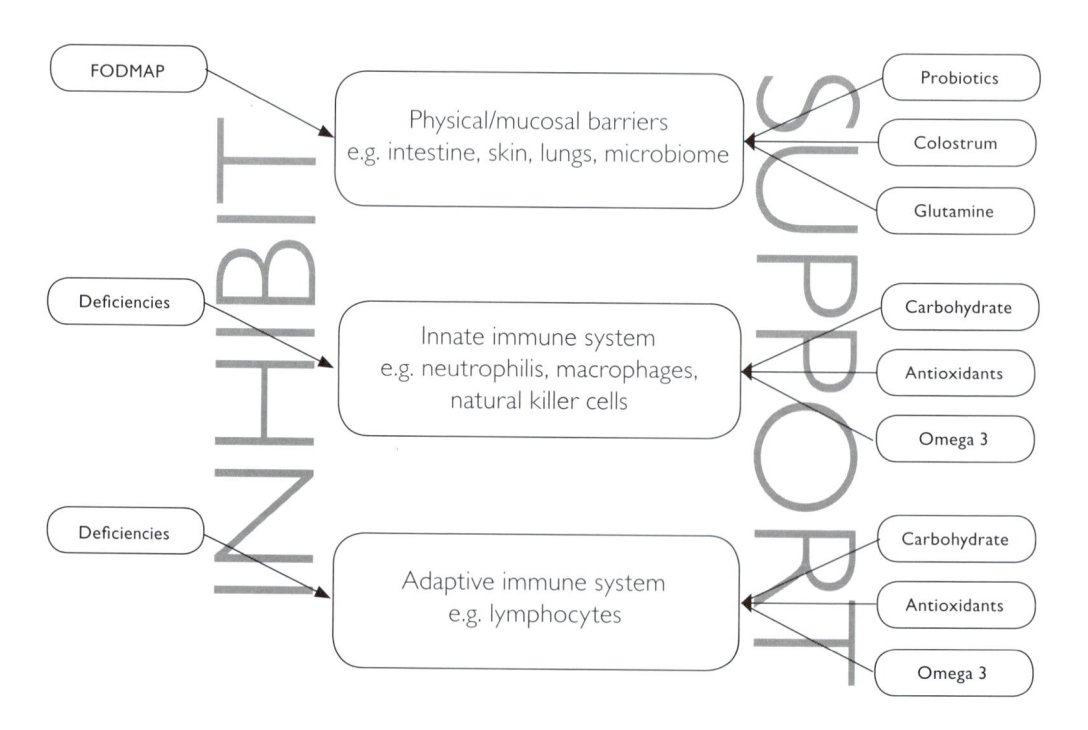

Nutritional influences on the immune system.

PREVENTING ILLNESS

Number of weeks during a sixteen-week intervention period where symptoms of an upper respiratory tract infection occurred with either probiotic (Pro) or placebo (Pla) supplementation (Gleeson et al., 2010).

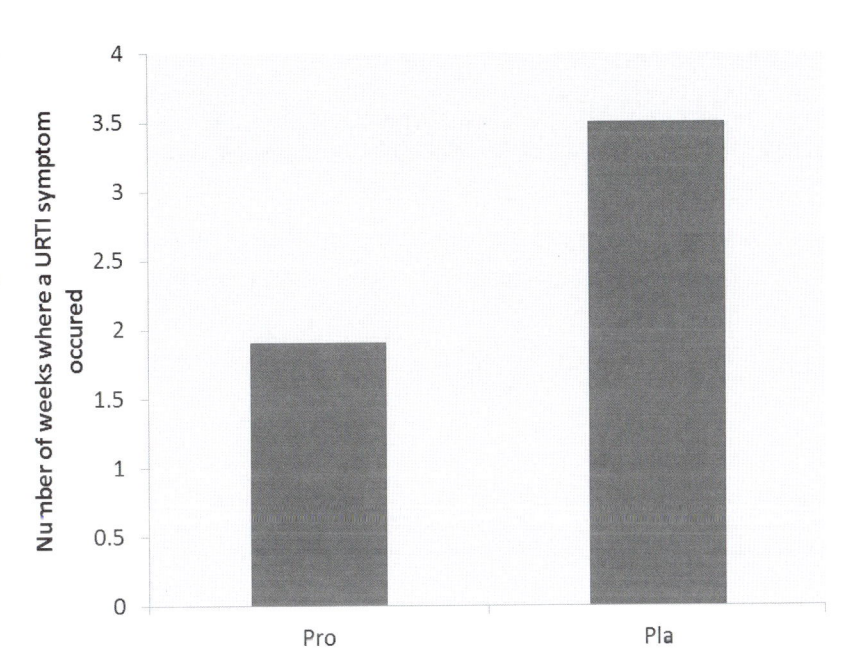

Gleeson et al. clearly showed that taking a probiotic yogurt twice per day reduced the incidence of illness. Quite significantly, too. The chances of getting an upper respiratory tract infection (a cold or sore throat in normal speak) was reduced by 36 per cent. This was matched by a significantly higher salivary IgA in the probiotic group. A lower salivary IgA has been linked to an increased risk of infection.

West et al. (2011) and Cox et al. (2010) also showed a reduction in illness with the use of a probiotic (this time *Lactobacillus fermentum*). Cox et al. showed a reduction in colds and sore throats, but the West et al. results were less conclusive. Although the results of West et al. did seem to demonstrate less illness in male athletes taking a probiotic, they showed some interesting results in female athletes that pointed to a trend towards an increase in illness. Alongside this, the male athletes showed a significant increase in the amount of *Lactobacillus fermentum* in the gut, but females did not. This starts to question how effective probiotics may be for female athletes.

The effects are also strain specific. Gleeson's group recently showed that supplementing with *Lactobacillus salivarius* had no effect on illness rates for athletes undertaking endurance training.

It seems that probiotics are useful for athletes to take, and they appear to cause minimal harm. However, the effect is specific to the strain taken and may also be gender specific too, with men seemingly getting more out of them.

Colostrum

Colostrum may be another nutritional product that influences the intestinal mucosa to reduce the incidence of illness in athletes. Colostrum is powdered milk obtained from a cow in the first forty-eight hours after giving birth to a calf. There is very little evidence that colostrum will directly impact exercise

PREVENTING ILLNESS

performance, or adaptation from training. However, in the last five to ten years there has been emerging evidence on the use of colostrum in reducing coughs and colds. A recent study from Aberystwyth University showed that just 20g of colostrum supplement per day could reduce the incidence of coughs and colds, particularly during high-risk

RESEARCH SPOTLIGHT

Probiotics and performance

There have been a handful of studies linking probiotic supplementation to health-based outcomes for athletes. However, in 2014 the first study was published which showed an effect on performance. A research group based in Australia, led by Cecilia Shing, looked at the effect of probiotic supplementation on exercise performance in the heat. Ten trained endurance runners undertook a supplementation period for four weeks, twice, separated by a three-week washout period. For the first time around half of the runners supplemented with 45 billion probiotic bacteria per day consisting of Lactobacillus, Bifidobacterium and Streptococcus strains. The other runners received a placebo. For the second four-week period the runners swapped over.

After each four-week period the runners exercised to fatigue at 80 per cent of their VO_2 max in 35°C heat and 40 per cent humidity. This is a considerable heat strain and will inhibit performance by itself. During these runs markers of intestinal permeability were measured. There were significant trends towards reductions in intestinal permeability and the absorption of toxins due to this reduced permeability. While statistical significance was not reached, there was a strong trend towards probiotics reducing the stress on the intestine due to exercise.

Of most interest, there was a significant increase in time to exhaustion due to probiotic supplementation. On average when probiotics had been supplemented there was a 16 per cent greater run time to exhaustion compared to placebo alone. As the first study to show an impact on exercise performance, the results may provide an interesting avenue to influence endurance performance.

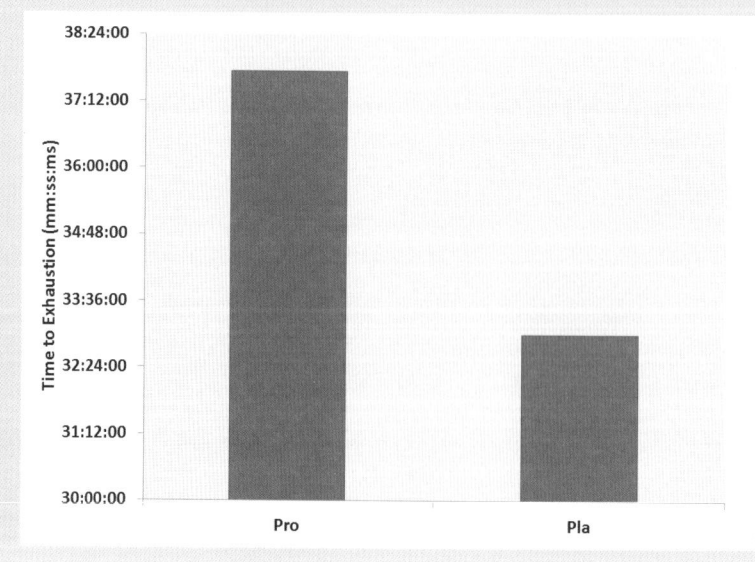

Run time to exhaustion following four weeks of probiotic or placebo supplementation (Shing et al., 2014).

PREVENTING ILLNESS

periods for illness such as the winter or high-volume training blocks. During such periods, this piece of research showed that 12 per cent of the subjects in the colostrum supplemented group suffered from a cough or cold. In the non-colostrum supplemented group 32 per cent of the participants got a cough or cold. This research is starting to be supported by others showing similar outcomes.

One of the potential mechanisms for reduction in illness through colostrum is through reducing intestinal permeability. If running is taken as an exercise model, then colostrum can reduce the increase in permeability post-exercise by up to 80 per cent.

It should be noted that colostrum is a controversial supplement. It contains naturally high amounts of the hormone IGF-1, which is on the World Anti-Doping Agency list of prohibited substances. However, research seems to suggest the IGF-1 is not absorbed when colostrum is consumed, even at very high doses of over 60g per day. Athletes should make themselves aware of any risks associated with colostrum before choosing to supplement with it.

Glutamine

Colostrum is not the only supplement that can reduce intestinal permeability. Glutamine is well known for doing this, too. Much of the research focus on glutamine has been as a direct fuel for the immune system, mostly coming from research into various clinical situations such as trauma. However, it is debatable as to whether taking glutamine during exercise has much impact on the immune system directly. It is more likely that glutamine will act on athletes by reducing intestinal permeability. There is some clinical research to suggest that this may be the case.

FOOD ALLERGIES

Many common food allergies that are given time in the press and in magazines do not really exist. There are many tests available that claim to tell you which foods you are allergic to and which are OK. However, none has any scientific validity and they should be avoided.

One potentially interesting development has been the role of FODMAP foods in the treatment of Inflammatory Bowel Disease (IBS). FODMAP stands for foods which contain Fermentable Oligo-Disaccarhides Mono Saccharides and Polyols. As you can see, FODMAP is far easier to pronounce.

These nutrients have been indicated to produce the symptoms of IBS in some people. When ingested, sugars such as fructose, lactose and fructans are osmotically active, causing water to move into the intestine and leading to luminal distention. Luminal distension can also be caused by fibrous sugars like galactans and polyols due to fermentation of the sugars in the intestine. Luminal distension can lead to bloating and pain as well as changes in stool production and wind.

Little research has been conducted on FODMAPs in athletes. However, this could be an interesting area to consider, especially for those who regularly suffer from gastrointestinal discomfort.

Carbohydrate

As we have seen, exercise puts intense pressure on the physical barriers of the immune system and on the infantry who stand behind it waiting to attack the invading hordes. Like all armies, a knight in shining armour is needed

PREVENTING ILLNESS

to succeed, and of course carbohydrate takes on the role in the interactions between exercise and the immune system.

Carbohydrate plays an important role in the immune system through two mechanisms. Firstly, maintaining blood glucose within the normal physiological range of 4–6mmol/l, and secondly by maintaining muscle glycogen stores. Blood glucose is the primary fuel for many aspects of the immune system, including the neutrophils and macrophages of the innate immune system or infantry, and those Special Forces of the acquired immune system, the lymphocytes. A decrease in blood glucose leads to a reduction in fuel for the immune system and therefore a compromise in function. For endurance exercise in particular it is common to see a reduction in blood glucose, thereby leading to a compromised immune system until this is restored. A reduction in muscle glycogen concentration can also trigger an inflammatory response, putting further strain on the immune system.

Muscle glycogen concentration is primarily determined by the exercise we undertake and the carbohydrate content of the diet. Even after two or three days of a low carbohydrate diet (less than 10 per cent of total energy intake) negative effects on the immune system can be seen. This is an important consideration for endurance athletes in particular.

The intake of simple carbohydrates during endurance exercise is well known to improve performance. However, there seems to be another benefit in terms of effects on the immune system. Simply ingesting 30–60g of

---

RESEARCH SPOTLIGHT

Timing and immunity

Many aspects of sports nutrition are influenced by the timing of nutrient intake. The influence of food and the immune system is no different. Ricardo Costa, then at Bangor University, investigated the effect of timing of carbohydrate and protein intake on a raft of immune markers. Nine male runners ran for two hours at 75 per cent VO_2 max on three occasions. One occasion, both immediately and one hour after exercise, the participants consumed only water; a second time they consumed 1.2g of carbohydrate per kilogram of body weight and 0.4g of protein per kilogram of body weight immediately after the run, and water an hour later. The final trial involved consuming water first, and then an hour later having the carbohydrate and protein drink.

For two hours and twenty minutes after the run various markers of immune function were measured. Many of them showed very little change. However, the response of one member of the tough infantry we have in place to attack invading hordes, the neutrophils, was different. When athletes consumed water only, or delayed their carbohydrate and protein intake by just one hour, there was a 24 per cent and 31 per cent decrease in their ability to release the toxins that attack the hordes. This process, called 'bacterially stimulated neutrophil degranulation', was not decreased at all when the carbohydrate and protein were consumed immediately after the run.

It can easily be seen how athletes might wait an hour before having food. By the time they have had a shower, maybe a quick conversation with their teammates or coach, an hour will fly by. The study from Costa and colleagues shows this may have a negative effect on their immune system and leave them open to infection and illness. The infantry will be weaker.

PREVENTING ILLNESS

Table 1.1 The role of vitamins and minerals in supporting the immune system.

Vitamin or Mineral	Role in the Immune System	Sources
Vitamin C	Acts as an antioxidant; increased amounts during coughs and colds may reduce the length of illness	Oranges, berries, broccoli, potatoes
Vitamin E	A fat-soluble vitamin, which also acts as an antioxidant	Nuts and seeds, fish, olives, broccoli
Zinc	Plays a role in many enzyme functions and reactions	Shellfish, nuts, red meat, wheat
Iron	Important in oxygen transports as a precursor of haemoglobin in red cells	Red meat, fish, green leafy vegetables
Copper	Deficiency alters the function of antioxidant defences such as selenium and glutathione	Shellfish, wholegrains, beans and lentils

Table 1.2 Food sources that are high in polyphenol, and effective daily dose to support the immune system.

Food	Serving Size
Dark chocolate (70% cocoa minimum)	40g
Red kidney beans	½ cup
Blueberries	1 cup
Blackberries	1½ cups
Strawberries	2 cups
Plums	3 plums
Red Delicious apples	3 apples
Raspberries	1 cup
Olives	1 handful
Spinach	1 handful
Walnuts	1 tablespoon chopped nuts
Green tea	1–2 cups
Green coffee	1–2 cups

17

PREVENTING ILLNESS

Table 1.3 Different types of fats in the diet and their role in the body.

Type of Fat	Role in the Body	Sources
Saturated fat	Often linked to development of chronic diseases such as cardiovascular disease. However, latest evidence may suggest not all are harmful	Cream, cheese, butter, red meat
Mono-unsaturated fats	Provides a potential source of energy. Have been linked to positive health outcomes	Olives, avocado, meat, milk, nuts
Polyunsaturated fats	Omega 3 and 6 fatty acids in particular have a role in inflammation and immunity. Increase the membrane fluidity of cells	Fish, nuts
Trans fats	Generally harmful for the body	Processed foods

carbohydrates during prolonged and intense exercise can reduce the negative effects of exercise on the immune system. However, when the exercise is of shorter duration or includes rest periods, the effect of carbohydrate during exercise is less clear. It is likely that where there is a risk of a reduction in blood glucose during exercise, consuming carbohydrates will prevent a drop in the effectiveness of the immune system.

Timing of carbohydrate intake also seems key. Just delaying the intake of carbohydrates by one hour can lead to a greater inhibition of the immune system than if the carbohydrates are taken on immediately post-exercise. It is commonplace for athletes to consume both carbohydrate and protein post-exercise. However, in terms of the immune system it is clear that the carbohydrate portions of these 'recovery' meals are the key component. The likely mechanism is maintenance of blood glucose and restoration of muscle glycogen concentration. As explained in Chapters 3 and 8, protein is important in the post-exercise recovery meal, but for other reasons.

Antioxidants and vitamins

Antioxidants and vitamins such as vitamin C and E could play a role in supporting the immune system. It is clear that deficiency in pretty much any nutrient will lead to a compromise of the immune system. However, there is very little evidence that nutrients can 'boost' the immune system, despite many claims being made.

In general, nutrients work in synergy within the body and any attempt to undo this balance can lead to compromised immunity. Therefore, many studies that have looked at boosting single nutrients tend not to show a positive effect. In some instances mega-dosing of single nutrients can lead to an inhibition of not only the immune system but the adaptive response to exercise. Caution should therefore be taken when looking to

PREVENTING ILLNESS

supplement with mega-doses of single nutrients.

Recently there has been a trend to investigate the effects of wholefoods on various immune variables. Cherry juice is one such example and has been shown to speed up the recovery of the immune system after hard exercise such as marathon running. This is most likely because of the presence of bioactive compounds called anthocyanins, which belong to the nutrient group termed polyphenols. It is likely that consuming good-quality, unprocessed foods will enable athletes to take in enough of the key antioxidants, vitamins and minerals to support their immune system.

Fat

Never has the saying 'You are what you eat' been more apt than for the function of fat in the body. You're probably thinking, of course that's the case: if you eat fat you get 'fat'. Well, it's not really. In reality fat plays an essential role in allowing the body to function effectively, as the fats we eat are incorporated into the structure of all the cells of the body. The different types of fat you eat influence the function of the cells in your body, and subsequently your body, in a number of ways. They influence how 'pliable' your cells are. The best example to give is that of the red blood cell. If you eat more omega 3 fatty acids, often found in oily fish such as salmon, then more of these are incorporated into the red blood cells, which makes them more pliable – meaning they find it easier to pass through the small capillaries they need to. However, if your diet is higher in omega 6 polyunsaturated fatty acids, then the red blood cell becomes more rigid, making it harder for it to pass through the small capillaries.

Omega 3 fatty acids also impact on the inflammatory response of a cell. The process is quite complicated, but imagine the type of fat incorporated into a cell as an amplifier. Some sort of stress reaction occurs inside the cell, and this is picked up by the amplifier as a signal. If the cell has a significant incorporation of omega 3 fatty acids, the signal is dampened; if the cell contains a significant amount of omega 6, the signal is amplified. This seemingly has an effect on the immune system, too. Although there is little exercise-specific research, research from clinical situations clearly shows the importance of omega 3 fatty acids in immunity, but also that too high an intake of omega 3 could actually be detrimental to the immune system. As always, too much of a good thing may not always be good.

Omega 6 fatty acids can be reduced in the diet by simply cutting out processed food, the most common source. Increasing omega 3 intake can also lead to an increase in omega 3 fatty acids incorporated into cells. Essentially the more omega 3 fatty acids you consume, the more is incorporated. Just consuming the equivalent of one portion of oily fish (e.g. salmon or mackerel) per week significantly increases the incorporation of omega 3 fatty acids into cells. If you can manage four portions per week, the incorporation is fourfold.

Summary

- Your immune system can be thought of as having three parts with which to defend itself from any foreign bodies trying to invade your body and do you harm.
- Firstly, the physical barriers such as your skin, and, more relevant to exercise and nutrition, the intestine. As you increase exercise duration, your intestine becomes more permeable, allowing easier passage

PREVENTING ILLNESS

of foreign bodies and increasing the risk of infection. The decrease in blood flow to the intestine with exercise also causes micro-damage, which furthers compromises function.
- The second line of defence is the innate immune system. This acts like the infantry of your body's defence system, and includes a variety of cells including neutrophils, macrophages and natural killer cells. Each have their own action, but in general they attack any invading body and are not specific.
- The final line of defence is the adaptive immune system, which acts like the Special Forces. They have memory for specific invaders; you may know them as your lymphocytes or antibodies.
- Both the innate and acquired immune system follow a similar pattern after exercise. There is at first an increase in the number of immune cells, followed by a decrease post-exercise. This is coupled with a decrease in function of the immune cells.

Gold
Preventing deficiencies: Long periods of starvation and/or dehydration can lead to a compromised immune system. Inadequate intake of protein, minerals such as copper, iron and zinc, or vitamins C and E can also compromise the immune system.

Carbohydrate intake during exercise: Where blood glucose may begin to decrease, supplementing with 30–60g of carbohydrate will prevent the decrease in immune function that is seen after exercise.

Timing of post-exercise carbohydrate: Consuming 1g per kg of body weight of carbohydrate immediately after intense or prolonged exercise, particularly where muscle glycogen concentration has been decreased, will support the immune system.

Silver
Probiotics: These have been shown to reduce the incidence of upper respiratory tract infections in athletes. Effects are strain specific, with evidence for *Lactobacillus casei* (shirota), and *Lactobacillus fermentum* in particular. Doses of 1.3×10^{11} and 1.0×10^9 respectively have been proven to reduce upper respiratory tract infections.

Colostrum: 10–20g of colostrum taken daily may provide defence against upper respiratory tract infections in athletes. Colostrum is the milk produced by mammals in the first few days after giving birth. Bovine colostrum is most commonly used in supplements.

Bronze
Glutamine: 5–10g daily of glutamine may help prevent any increase in intestinal permeability. However, this has not been shown to reduce illness in athletes.

FODMAPs: Some evidence in clinical situations for the treatment of IBS-type conditions. Limited evidence in exercise situations.

Polyphenols: A good theoretical research base to support supplementation of foods such as cherry juice. However, limited evidence to support their use, and in some cases may also inhibit the adaptation to training. Choosing foods high in polyphenols is recommended where possible.

Omega 3 fats: More commonly known as fish oils. These have a theoretical role in supporting the immune system when a dose of 1–2g per day is taken. However, there is currently little evidence to support their use. Food

PREVENTING ILLNESS

Table 1.4 Example diet plan for Chapter 1.

Meal	Food
Breakfast	Bowl of porridge with semi-skimmed milk, with raspberries and walnuts 1 Greek yogurt 1 probiotic yogurt 1 apple Glass of juice Cup of tea with milk
Snack during a two-hour cycle ride	2 bananas, 2 carbohydrate gels and 1 bottle of carbohydrate drink
Lunch	Egg mayonnaise sandwich on white bread Fruit corner yogurt 1 can of cola
Snack	1 bar of chocolate 1 medium latte
Dinner	Oven-roast chicken breast with oven chips, a green salad with salad cream dressing Ice cream for dessert

Carbohydrate (g/kg body weight) 4.2	Protein (g/kg body weight) 1.2	Fat (g/kg body weight) 1.2

sources of omega 3, such as oily fish, should be promoted where possible.

Further reading

Costa, R. J. S., Oliver, S. J., Laing, S. J., Walters, R., Bilzon, J. L. J. & Walsh, N. P. (2009). Influence of timing of post-exercise carbohydrate-protein ingestion on selected immune indices. *International Journal of Sport Nutrition and Exercise Metabolism*, 19(4), 366–84.

Gleeson, M., Bishop, N. C., Oliveira, M., & Tauler, P. (2011). Daily Probiotics (*Lactobacillus casei* Shirota) Reduction of Infection Incidence in Athletes. *International Journal of Sport Nutrition*, (2010), 55–64.

Gleeson, M., Bishop, N.C., Walsh, N.P. (2013). *Exercise Immunology*. Elsevier Press.

Shing, C. M., Peake, J. M., Lim, C. L., Briskey, D., Walsh, N. P., Fortes, M. B., Vitetta, L. (2014). Effects of probiotics supplementation on gastrointestinal permeability, inflammation and exercise performance in the heat. *European Journal of Applied Physiology*, 114(1), 93–103.

VanHeest, J. L., Rodgers, C. D., Mahoney, C. E. & De Souza, M. J. (2014). Ovarian suppression impairs sport performance in junior elite female swimmers. *Medicine and Science in Sports and Exercise*, 46(1), 156–66.

CHAPTER 2

NUTRITION FOR INJURY

Injuries can cause frustration and pain for athletes. They can lead to significant time out of their sport, and in some cases can end a career. Over the last ten years or so the role of food in injury prevention and treatment has started to become apparent, particularly for those niggling annoying injuries caused by overuse, like a stress fracture or a muscle tear. Let's start with the most basic aspect of nutrition to influence injury: how much energy you consume.

Energy availability

Exercise needs energy, as does your body to go about its daily function. If energy needs when exercising keep going up, and this increase in energy use is not counteracted by taking on board more energy, the body begins to get into trouble.

The best way to describe what happens when not enough energy is consumed is to look at the female athlete. Here we find the female athlete triad: the interaction of low energy availability, menstrual dysfunction and bone health.

Let's begin with energy availability, which is the energy left for the body to perform bodily functions after the energy cost of exercise has been removed. It is different from being in energy balance. It is defined as energy intake minus the energy needed for the exercise performed divided by the amount of lean body mass in kg (kcal/kgLBM/day).

On average, when in energy balance, females have an energy availability of 40 kcal/kgLBM/day. Here physiological function is normal, menstrual function will be normal barring any other complications, and bone health will be normal.

Let's take our female in energy balance and add in some exercise training, and make an assumption that energy intake is not increased to match this. Incidentally, this is very common. Just because we start to exercise, doesn't mean that we eat more. This seems especially so in females; males seem to more easily increase their energy intake in response to exercise.

So our female athlete's energy availability has decreased to 30 kcal/kgLBM/day. Here we start to see some small physiological changes; these aren't significant but give us an indication of what is to come. Circulating concentrations of the hormones IGF-1 and triiodothyronine (T3), a thyroid hormone, start to decrease. These two hormones are sensitive to energy availability, and it seems likely that the decrease in IGF-1 is a consequence of the decrease in T3. T3 has potent effects on nearly every part of the human body and plays a role in growth and energy metabolism. However, at 30 kcal/kgLBM/day these decreases in hormones have only a small physiological effect. Bone should still be fine, as should the menstrual cycle, along with the hormonal responses associated with it.

So now our female athlete has been exer-

NUTRITION FOR INJURY

cising a while. She decides she should lose some weight and reduces her calorie intake. All of a sudden her energy availability is only 20 kcal/kgLBM/day. T3 and IGF-1 begin to fall rapidly. Both of these hormones have potent effects on the bone. T3 and IGF-1 both stimulate bone formation. As energy availability drops below 30 kcal/kgLBM/day we start to see significant reductions in markers of bone formation.

Our female athlete continues her weight-loss plan; energy availability is still at 20 kcal/kgLBM/day. Now we start to see effects on hormones related to the menstrual cycle. Luteinizing hormone (LH) is a hormone that is frequently pulsed, particularly around menstruation. This pulsing is key, with normal function looking like small and frequent surges. In our female athlete with a decreased energy availability, these pulses will be larger and less frequent.

It is likely that our female athlete may be suffering from some menstrual dysfunction now. Her periods will be becoming irregular. She is also more likely to get bone injuries as bone formation has started to become compromised.

Let's assume our athlete has not got injured. She is training well, and losing weight. Performance is improving; she has just set a new personal best. This loss in body weight is really helping her performance. She decides to up her training a little, and cut out a bit more food. Now her energy availability is 10 kcal/kgLBM/day.

As you can imagine, T3 and IGF-1 continue

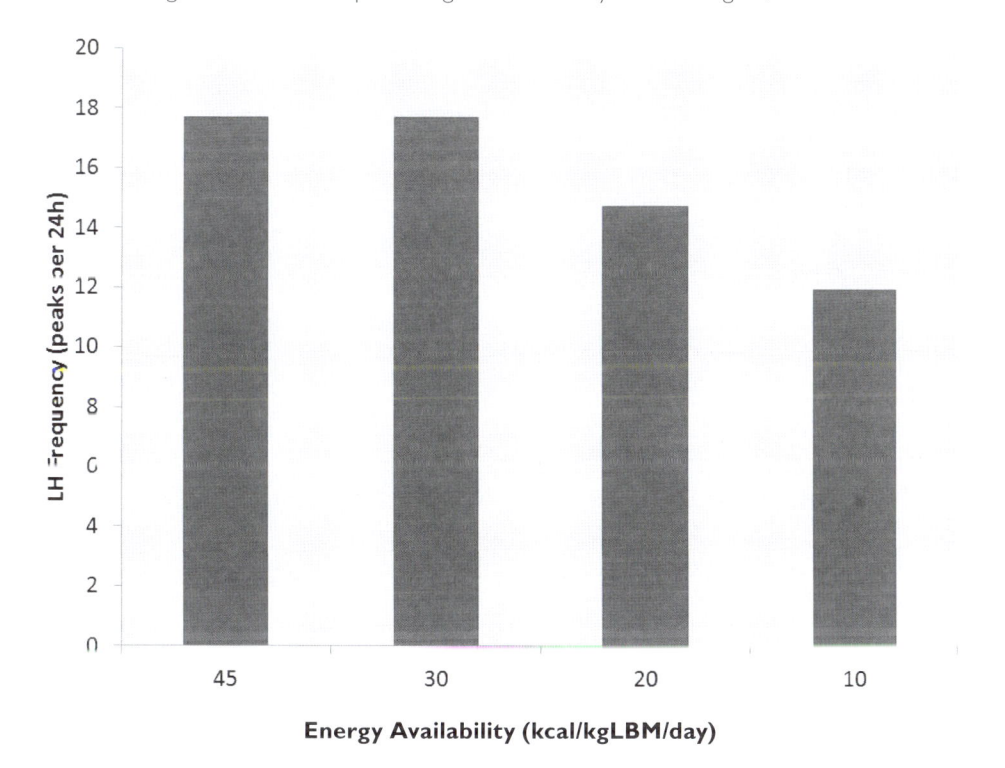

Luteinizing hormone frequency over a 24-hour period at different energy availabilities (adapted from Loucks and Thuma, 2003).

NUTRITION FOR INJURY

to fall, although not as dramatically as before. LH continues to pulse, but the peaks become even higher and less frequent. Her menstrual function is highly likely to have become irregular or non-existent. The final nail in the coffin is her bones. The production of oestrogen now becomes suppressed, and a decrease in oestrogen production leads to an increase in bone resorption, or bone breakdown.

Now we have the perfect storm for bone. Energy availability has decreased to such a degree that bone formation has decreased and bone breakdown has increased. This athlete is on a one-way street to getting a stress fracture. More recent research, mainly in animals, has shown that a reduction in oestrogen production can also increase rates of tendon breakdown, increasing the risk of tendon injuries, one of the most common injuries for athletes.

Taken together, it can be seen that as far as the female athlete is concerned, decreasing the energy available for the body to perform normal functions will lead to a significantly higher risk of an injury occurring. This is likely

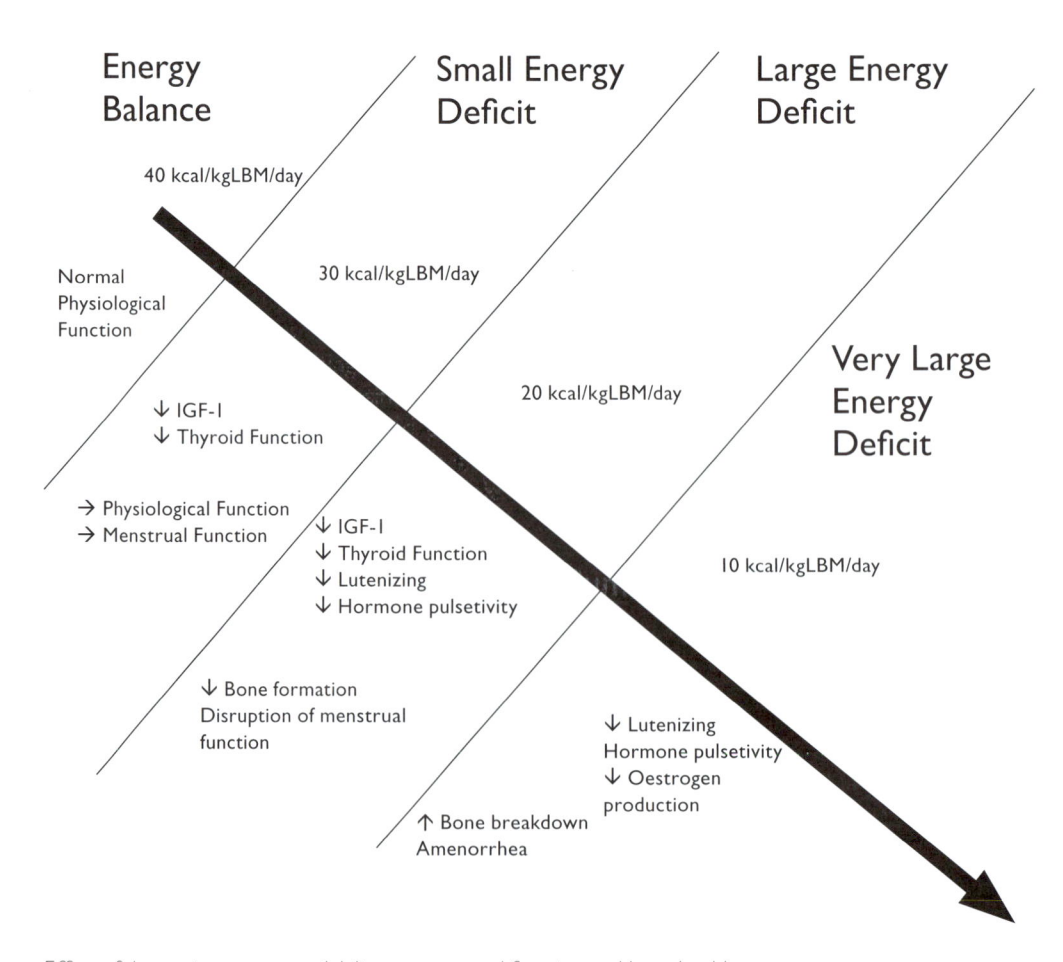

Effect of decreasing energy availability on menstrual function and bone health.

NUTRITION FOR INJURY

to be similar for men too, except that it is testosterone which is decreased, not oestrogen. Far more research has been conducted in females than males in this area.

The original concept of the female athlete triad was linked to eating disorders. Of course, eating disorders will lead to a decrease in energy availability. However, a decrease in energy availability does not automatically indicate an eating disorder. Often it is a lack of nutrition education and understanding that occurs.

In the scenario of our female athlete we also saw the high risk of linking performance to body weight. She saw a decrease in body weight and linked it to an increase in performance. This will be covered in more depth in Chapter 10, but is often a vicious circle that particularly affects endurance runners.

Muscle tear

You're through on goal, legs running at full speed. Past the last defender. Just the goalkeeper to beat. Just a few more strides before the ball can be struck. Then all of a sudden a twinge occurs at the back of the hamstring. One more stride, the twinge becomes agony, the knee won't bend any more. The defender sneaks in and takes the ball off your toes. Meanwhile you crumple to the floor, your hamstring unable to work any longer. There is a tear in the hamstring.

At this point the pain will be bad. Within the muscle itself, the body will be kicking into action. The infantry we met in the last chapter will be entering the damaged muscle tissue. The macrophages will be working to break down the damaged tissue. This process can take up to three days and is an essential part of the process to kick-start repair.

During the process of necrosis, an inflammatory response will start, followed by an anti-inflammatory response. At this point the regeneration process kicks into overdrive, with the proliferation of satellite cells within the muscle. Satellite cells are precursors to muscle cells. Think of them as baby muscle cell eggs waiting to be fertilized. The inflammatory process essentially fertilizes these baby muscle cells and starts their growth process.

As these satellite cells within muscle divide and grow they form new muscle cells, which can then replace those that were damaged when the muscle was torn. However, there is a competitor at this point and that is connective tissue. Where possible the muscle fibre should regrow fully; however, sometimes scarring occurs in the tissue, forcing connective tissue to grow instead of muscle tissue.

How does nutrition play a role in this? Firstly, we need to provide the building blocks to rebuild the damaged muscle. These building blocks are proteins. A regular intake of high-quality proteins on a daily basis will provide the building blocks to repair the damaged muscle. Protein should be consumed every three to four hours during the day to provide a constant supply of building blocks. Proteins high in the amino acid leucine should be chosen where possible; this should begin early in the process of injury.

Foods high in leucine:

- cottage cheese
- lentils
- fish (particularly tuna and cod)
- peanuts
- almonds
- meat
- dairy foods
- whey protein

About three days after the injury occurs the nutrients consumed can influence satellite

NUTRITION FOR INJURY

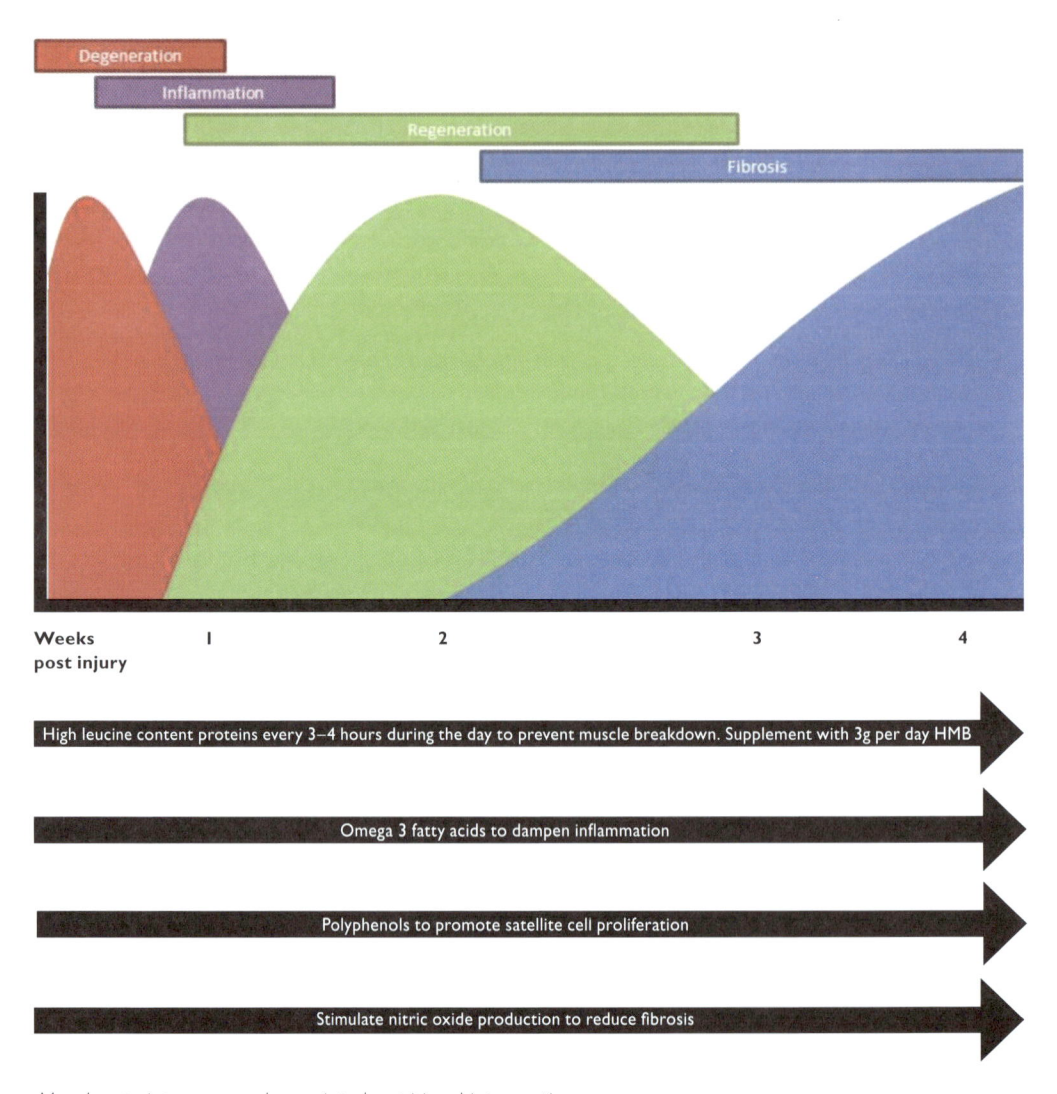

Muscle repair process and associated nutritional interventions.

cell proliferation. Foods high in polyphenols should be consumed as these have been shown to promote satellite cell proliferation and speed up the healing process in muscle post-injury. Foods such as berries should be considered (see Table 1.2 for a list of foods).

About ten days post-injury there is an opportunity to promote muscle fibre regeneration and prevent muscle scarring. At this point nitric oxide plays a role in favouring muscle regeneration over scarring. Nutrients such as arginine, citrulline and dietary nitrates can influence nitric oxide and should be considered at this point in the rehabilitation process.

NUTRITION FOR INJURY

Foods high in dietary nitrates:

- celery
- cress
- chervil
- lettuce
- beetroot
- spinach
- rocket
- Swiss chard

Bone fractures

The hamstring tear was annoying, you were out for a few weeks, but with good nutrition there was always the chance you would get back more quickly. Your physio has given you the all-clear to start training again. You quickly get back into the swing of things, and increase the training load. There is a big Cup Final only six weeks away, and if you can just increase the amount of training you do then maybe, just maybe, you can make the team.

You're a few weeks into the training, when during a run you feel a sharp ache in your foot. You better get it checked out. The physio pulls a strained face. Her brow lifts. Her forehead wrinkles. A frown appears. She shakes her head. She sends you for a scan. The results are back. A stress fracture has occurred: the consequence of the increased training load.

It is known that changes in training load, in particular a step change in training volume, can lead to an increased risk of stress fractures. Bone is not just a solid lump of matter, it is metabolically active, and continually goes through a process of formation and resorption (breakdown). Bone is made up of organic compounds, primarily in the form of collagen, which is the structural protein of connective tissue. These organic compounds make up approximately 40 per cent of the bone's structure. The other 60 per cent of the bone is made of inorganic compounds, primarily the mineral calcium.

Obviously, as an increase in training volume occurs, sheer mechanical stress can itself lead to a stress fracture, especially in combination with poor technique or equipment, such as running shoes. The other aspect is the biological effects of exercise on bone.

As you go out for long runs, exhaustion will inevitably occur with glycogen depletion. And if you went for that run but then didn't exercise for four days, you would see an increase in bone breakdown over those four days. However, there would not be a similar increase in bone formation. Therefore, an imbalance is caused where bone breakdown outstrips bone formation.

Of course, you are likely to train again in this timeframe. What you will see is that while the acute increase in bone breakdown is suppressed, there is a general elevation in bone breakdown without an increase in bone formation following it. However, if you increase exercise intensity, there is no further effect on bone breakdown or formation.

So how does nutrition interact with exercise to influence bone metabolism? As we saw at the beginning of the chapter, reducing energy intake has significant negative effects on bone, primarily through hormonal changes in the body affecting both bone formation and breakdown. Certainly, male and female athletes who underconsume food are going to face a significant risk of stress fracture.

Underconsumption of calcium in the diet is also a significant risk factor for stress fractures. This is no surprise, as calcium is a major contributor to bone structure. There is considerable research in young female athletes, which has shown that increasing calcium intake over 1000mg per day leads to a decreased risk of stress fractures throughout their life. Calcium absorption is regulated by vitamin D.

NUTRITION FOR INJURY

> **VITAMIN D – A NUTRIENT WITH MANY ROLES**
>
> Vitamin D has received much attention over the last few years as an important nutrient for many reasons, not least sports performance. Let's start with a disclaimer. In reality very little vitamin D is consumed via food. While there is some in foods such as eggs, and it is often added to foods via a fortification process, the amounts found are not sufficient. Often, in order to reach sufficient intakes, supplementation needs to be in place.
>
> Our bodies have evolved to synthesize vitamin D through exposure to sunlight. Certainly, those countries that have a lower exposure to sunlight – those in the northern hemisphere in particular – show a higher prevalence of vitamin D deficiency. While vitamin D was originally thought of as a nutrient, it might be more accurate to think of it as a hormone than as a vitamin.
>
> There is increasing evidence of deficiency across various populations, which could be due to a variety of reasons, from a lack of exposure to sunlight through to dietary fat intake. However, a deficiency in vitamin D does have some consequences on how the body functions. Recent evidence suggests that reductions in vitamin D increase the risks of upper respiratory tract infections, increase the risk of injury and reduce muscle function.
>
> A deficiency in vitamin D can have significant effects on bone in particular. Vitamin D is essential in the process of absorption for calcium, along with other nutrients such as iron. Calcium is constantly being turned over within bone and if there is insufficient calcium available bone breakdown will ensue. If athletes are deficient in vitamin D, they are at a higher risk of stress fractures in particular.
>
> Vitamin D status can be easily monitored through measurement of serum 25 hydroxyvitamin D concentrations. There are a number of recommendations for appropriate concentrations for health and wellbeing. However, generally a score less than 30 nmol/l is seen as deficient, 30–75 nmol/l as insufficient, with an optimal range somewhere in the range of 75–150 nmol/l, with concerns of going higher than this due to a higher risk of toxicity.
>
> So if an athlete is deficient in vitamin D, what is the process to increase this? The European Food Standards Agency has recommended a highest dose of 4000 IU per day to restore insufficiency. If in any doubt, athletes should consult their medical team.

One of the most controversial areas around nutrition and bone is the impact of protein. Traditionally, it is thought that protein has a negative effect on bone health, leading to an increase in bone breakdown. This view suggests that protein leads to an acidic environment in the body, whereby the body tries to neutralize the acid by releasing calcium from the bone.

However, more recent evidence seems to suggest that this is not true. Research is now suggesting that increasing protein intake in periods of calorie deficit actually spares bone from breaking down. It certainly seems that protein has positive effects on bone, especially when matched with appropriate calcium intake and a high consumption of fruit and vegetables.

Other aspects of nutrition and bone come from correlational studies in post-menopausal women, who have a higher risk of osteoporosis. This evidence seems to suggest a role for vegetable intake in preventing bone loss, along with calcium and omega 3 fatty acids. Negative effects on bone can be seen with high intakes of alcohol and potentially caffeine, too.

Much of sports nutrition is based around the timing of food intake. Bone seems to be no different. Exercising in the fasted state leads to an increase in bone breakdown, but does not affect bone formation. If you consume

NUTRITION FOR INJURY

any macronutrient, bone breakdown will be decreased for three or four hours after the food has been ingested. Again, this is a similar timeframe to what you see in other parts of the body, such as muscle.

There is also some evidence that post-exercise food intake has an effect on bone breakdown. Delaying carbohydrate and protein intake by only one hour leads to a greater increase in markers of bone breakdown compared to taking on board the same meal immediately post-exercise. Calcium intake before and after training also seems to reduce the increase in bone breakdown seen with exercise.

Tendon injuries

Tendons are the connection between bone and muscle. Tendons are made up of approximately 85 per cent collagen, with the rest made up of various minerals. Tendon injury is common in many sports, as tendons are the conduit through which muscles apply force to bones to move the body. Taking a very broad brush approach, tendon injuries can be thought of in two types: rupture and tendinopathy. Ruptures are essentially a tear in the tendon to some degree, and tendinopathy is chiefly chronic pain.

So how can nutrition influence tendon health? At the most basic level the nutrients needed to build tendons can help repair a rupture. The major amino acids found in tendon collagen are proline and glycine. Both are pretty common in the diet, but are particularly high in foods such as chicken and gelatine. There is increasing evidence that supplementing with collagen itself can promote tendon healing and repair.

One feature of tendons is that blood flow is generally poor around them, leading to difficulties in supplying adequate nutrients.

Nitric oxide is a signalling molecule produced by the body that has multiple functions, one of which is to promote blood flow through capillaries. There is also the possibility of increasing tendon repair directly. A number of potential nutrients can promote nitric oxide formation:

- Dietary nitrates: These have been shown to increase nitric oxide formation and lead to an increase in blood flow. They can be found in foods such as beetroot and Swiss chard.
- Arginine: 8g of arginine per day has been shown to increase nitric oxide production. Alongside this, there is a potential of arginine stimulating growth hormone production, which will promote tendon healing.
- Citrulline malate: Another precursor of nitric oxide production. 8g per day seems to promote nitric oxide production.

The amino acid leucine appears to directly stimulate tendon formation. While evidence has appeared in mouse models of leucine promoting tendon formation, little is available in humans. However, a recent study has shown that when ingestion of 20g of whey protein, a protein naturally high in the leucine, was given immediately after exercise over a twelve-week training programme, there was a 15 per cent increase in tendon size, compared to only 8 per cent without the whey protein supplement.

Tendinopathies occur regularly in athletes. The same nutrition as that for a tendon rupture can also help a tendinopathy. Alongside this, two interventions have been shown to decrease the pain caused by a tendinopathy: firstly, omega 3 fatty acid supplementation of around 1–2g per day and, secondly, polyphenols. What is promising is that these two nutrients can work in

NUTRITION FOR INJURY

synergy with each other and physiotherapy to reduce the pain associated with a tendinopathy.

Maintaining muscle mass

No matter what type of injury you get, there is a good chance you will go through a period of doing limited or no training. It could even mean bed rest. A consequence of bed rest or inactivity is a loss of muscle mass. This is a threat to an athlete's ability to return to training quickly and performing again. What you eat at this point can be crucial to maintaining as much muscle mass as possible.

Once the injury occurs, speed is of the essence as the first couple of weeks after a limb, or the whole body, is immobilized is the time when most muscle mass is lost. During this time period muscle mass is lost at a rate of 0.5 per cent per day. It is possible that in highly trained athletes this rate of muscle mass loss is greater, as they will generally start with a greater amount of muscle than a sedentary person.

The loss of muscle mass associated with immobilization is not the only thing the athlete needs to worry about. The loss of muscle strength decreases at a rate approximately three times more quickly than muscle mass.

What you eat has a bearing on the loss of muscle due to immobilization. The most important factor is protein ingestion. Muscle is in a constant state of flux between being built up and broken down. With immobilization it seems that muscle protein synthesis, or build-up, is decreased, but breakdown stays the same. Therefore, there is an imbalance in favour of muscle protein breakdown.

To make things a little more complicated, the response of muscle protein synthesis to protein feeding is inhibited, and a state of anabolic resistance ensues. This is likely to be because of the decrease in muscle contractions due to immobilization. This anabolic resistance means there is an increased need for protein intake, as the amount of protein needed to stimulate muscle protein synthesis is increased. Normally, the amount of protein needed to stimulate muscle protein synthesis is 0.3g/kg of body weight per serving. However, when immobilized, this increases to 0.4g/kg of body weight per serving.

Increasing protein intake to 0.4g/kg of body weight per serving every three or four hours will also decrease any sensations of hunger that an athlete may feel. This will hopefully prevent overconsumption of other nutrients, which may not be needed during injury.

Protein content in the diet is the priority to prevent muscle mass loss during immobilization. However, there are also three supplements that are worth exploring:

- The first is β-hydroxy β-methylbutyrate (HMB), which is a metabolite of the amino acid leucine. There is some evidence that 3g per day of HMB can prevent loss of muscle mass during immobilization. Over a ten-day period of bed rest 3g of HMB, split into two doses of 1.5g per day, can decrease muscle mass loss by two-thirds.
- The second is omega 3 fatty acids. These are commonly found in fish, and consequently fish oil supplements. Supplementing with 4g per day of fish oil appears to reverse the anabolic resistance to protein seen with immobilization.
- Finally, creatine supplementation also appears to spare muscle mass during inactivity. While the evidence is not conclusive, 20g of creatine per day for five days at the beginning of immobilization appears to reduce the amount of muscle lost during immobilization.

NUTRITION FOR INJURY

Summary

- Ensuring the body has enough energy available to go about its daily functions is essential for injury prevention.
- Energy availability is the energy left after the energy cost of exercise has been removed. It is measured in kcal per kilogram of lean body mass per day (kcal/kgLBM/day).
- Female athletes when in energy balance have an energy availability of 40 kcal/kg LBM/day.
- Decreases in circulating concentrations of the hormones IGF-1 and triiodothyronine (T3) start to decrease at 30 kcal/kgLBM/day.
- At 20 kcal/kgLBM/day significant reductions in IGF-1 and T3 are observed. These start to influence bone formation. Subsequent to this, decreases in luteinizing hormone (LH) pulsatility occur, disrupting menstrual cycle function.
- Further reductions to 10 kcal/kgLBM/day lead to a reduction in circulating oestrogens and an increase in bone breakdown.
- It can be seen that consuming adequate energy is imperative for athletes to maintain bone function, and potentially tendon function too.
- Muscle tears are a common injury. After the injury has occurred, the muscle goes through a series of processes to ensure the muscle repairs itself. Firstly, an inflammatory response is triggered, which will work to break down the damaged tissue. Following this stage is a regeneration stage, where the satellite cells in the muscle begin to divide and grow into new muscle cells to replace those damaged during the injury.
- Bone is made up of approximately 40 per cent organic compounds such as collagen and 60 per cent inorganic compounds, with the largest being calcium. Increases in training volume or impact increase the risk of a stress fracture occurring in athletes.
- Tendons connect bones to muscle, and are an essential part of the musculoskeletal system. Nutrients can influence prevention of tendon injuries, as well as repair once injured.
- Maintaining muscle mass during periods of inactivity due to injury is essential for athletes. Muscle mass decreases at a rate of approximately 0.5 per cent per day during periods of inactivity.

Gold

Regular protein intake with muscle repair: Adequate protein intake will stimulate satellite cell formation and enhance muscle repair. Aim for 0.3g per kg of body weight every three to four hours.

Calcium for bone: Sufficient calcium intake is essential for strong healthy bones. The Recommended Daily Allowance for calcium is 700mg. This should be the minimum consumed through dietary sources for those who are undertaking exercise.

Vitamin D for bone: Athletes should be aiming for sufficiency in vitamin D. A blood test can help guide the need for individuals. Insufficient vitamin D influences calcium metabolism and therefore bone health.

Protein intake to maintain muscle mass: Aim for a serving size of 0.4g of protein per kg of body weight every three or four hours to minimize muscle mass loss during periods of inactivity.

Silver

Polyphenol intake to repair muscle: Three days post-injury is the optimal time to begin

NUTRITION FOR INJURY

increasing food high in polyphenols to further promote satellite cell proliferation.

Protein for bone: Protein does not seem to negatively influence bone in healthy exercising individuals. In periods of low energy availability sufficient protein intake, especially from dairy sources, may have a protective effect on bone.

Whey protein for tendons: Whey protein has a high, naturally occurring concentration of the amino acid leucine, which has a direct influence on tendons. Consuming 20g of whey protein after resistance exercise will strengthen tendons.

Bronze

Nitrate intake for muscle repair: Ten days after the injury occurs, dietary nitrates should be increased to promote nitric oxide formation. This will favour muscle regeneration over muscle scarring.

Nitric oxide for tendon: Dietary intake of nitrates and arginine influence the production of nitric oxide, which appears to be important for tendon health.

Omega 3 fatty acids for muscle mass: 1–2g of omega 3 fatty acids per day may help prevent loss of muscle during periods of inactivity.

Table 2.1 Example diet plan for Chapter 2.

Meal	Food
Breakfast	Large bowl of porridge made with semi-skimmed milk, with walnuts and raspberries, topped with 125g of Greek yogurt 1 apple 1 probiotic yogurt 1 cup of tea with milk
During exercise	2 bananas, 1 isotonic carbohydrate gel and 750ml of 6% carbohydrate electrolyte drink
Post-exercise	20g of whey protein with 35g of carbohydrates 1 apple
Lunch	1 tin of tuna with a baked sweet potato and a mixed salad
Snack	2 slices of wholemeal bread with almond butter
Post-exercise	1 pint of semi-skimmed milk made into a smoothie with blueberries
Dinner	1 chicken breast with brown rice, broccoli, kale and carrots
Pre-bed snack	1 orange

Carbohydrate (g/kg body weight)	Protein (g/kg body weight)	Fat (g/kg body weight)
5.9	2.1	1

HMB: Supplementation with 3g per day of HMB may help prevent loss of muscle during inactivity.

Creatine: Some evidence that 20g per day of creatine for five days may help prevent loss of muscle mass during inactivity.

Further reading

Farup, J., Rahbek, S. K., Knudsen, I. S., de Paoli, F., Mackey, A. L. & Vissing, K. (2014). Whey protein supplementation accelerates satellite cell proliferation during recovery from eccentric exercise. *Amino Acids*.

Gharaibeh, B., Chun-Lansinger, Y., Hagen, T., Ingham, S. J. M., Wright, V., Fu, F. & Huard, J (2012). Biological approaches to improve skeletal muscle healing after injury and disease. Birth Defects Research. Part C, *Embryo Today : Reviews*, 96(1), 82–94.

Kruger, M. J., & Smith, C. (2012). Postcontusion polyphenol treatment alters inflammation and muscle regeneration. *Medicine and Science in Sports and Exercise*. 44(5), 872–80.

Loucks, A. & Thuma J. (2003). Luteinizing hormone pulsatility is disrupted at a threshold of energy availability in regularly menstruating women. *Journal of Clinical Endocrinology and Metabolism*. 88 (1). 297-311.

Mountjoy, M., Sundgot-Borgen, J., Burke, L., Carter, S., Constantini, N., Lebrun, C., Ljungqvist, A. (2014). The IOC consensus statement: beyond the Female Athlete Triad–Relative Energy Deficiency in Sport (RED-S). *British Journal of Sports Medicine*, 48(7), 491–7.

Wall, B. T., Morton, J. P., & van Loon, L. J. C. (2014). Strategies to maintain skeletal muscle mass in the injured athlete: Nutritional considerations and exercise mimetics. *European Journal of Sport Science*, 1–10.

CHAPTER 3

USING NUTRITION TO MAXIMIZE ADAPTATION TO STRENGTH TRAINING

Sports nutrition faces a great challenge. It is the challenge of the magic bullet: the idea that taking a single pill or powder will automatically lead to a greater outcome, in some cases without training. Nowhere is this more evident than in the area of strength development and increases in muscle mass.

Nutrition acts as a facilitator for training adaptation. Without the training stimulus adaptation cannot occur. However, put the right nutrients into the body at the right time, and the training effect can be truly magnified. Over the coming chapter the nutrients that can be used to maximize the adaptive response to strength training will be outlined. Remember, though, there is no one single magic bullet. The training comes first, the nutrition second, but together they can create magic.

Fuelling

Carbohydrate. It's a dirty word, isn't it? Especially for strength and power athletes. It's only the endurance guys and girls who need carbohydrates. This appears not to be the case, however. Given certain types of resistance training, muscle glycogen stores can be decreased by up to 40 per cent. This is, however, dependent on the type of training performed. Hypertrophy-type strength training, where there is a high number of reps, at high intensity, has the greatest effect on muscle glycogen.

Significant decreases in muscle glycogen content can inhibit the force the muscle produces, and therefore reduce the effectiveness of the training session. This may lead over time to smaller gains in strength and muscle mass than originally planned and expected.

As a result of this, it is important in both the pre-exercise and post-exercise feeds to include a source of carbohydrate. Aiming for 1g/kg of body weight one to two hours prior to the training session, followed up by a further 1g/kg of body weight of carbohydrate immediately post-training, will maximize muscle glycogen status and therefore improve performance in the gym. The pre-training meal carbohydrates should consist of slow-release carbohydrate such as sweet potato or quinoa. The post-training meal should consist of quick-release carbohydrates such as those found in fruit.

Creatine

Click your fingers. Wait a minute. Click them

USING NUTRITION TO MAXIMIZE ADAPTATION TO STRENGTH TRAINING

again. Wait a minute. Click them again. Within the muscles you just used to click your fingers something incredible was happening. Those muscles were producing large amounts of force, in a fraction of a second. To create that energy to produce the high force, the body wasn't using carbohydrate or fat or protein as it normally would. It was using phosphocreatine. This is a high energy source found within muscle that can produce a lot of energy very quickly. However, stores of phosphocreatine are low and expire very quickly when in use. Your body can resynthesize them, and hence one minute later you can click your fingers again without even knowing your body has done anything. Try doing the same thing again, but keep going. Keep clicking your fingers constantly. How long did you last? Not too long would be my guess, due to waning phosphocreatine stores.

What if you could increase the levels of phosphocreatine within the muscle? Could you click your fingers more forcefully, more often? Creatine is a peptide made from the amino acids L-arginine, glycine and L-methionine, and is naturally synthesized in the body within the liver. Ninety five per cent of creatine found in the human body is found in muscle, and in a 70kg male there will be around 120g of creatine stored at any given time.

If you want to keep clicking your fingers, will supplementing with creatine help? I guess the first question that always needs to be asked when thinking about a supplement is can the ingredient, in this case creatine, be absorbed? Absorption of creatine monohydrate is around about 100 per cent absorption through the intestine. This is the first tick in the box. As an aside, there are many claims around different forms of creatine being better absorbed than creatine monohydrate. Yet it is hard to see how there can be any improvement in 100 per cent absorption. Therefore, creatine monohydrate is the most cost-effective way to get creatine into the body. Once creatine monohydrate has been ingested, peak blood concentrations of creatine occur within the hour.

Once creatine is absorbed it circulates in the blood until it reaches muscle. Here, creatine faces a challenge. It must pass through the cell wall of the muscle to get inside. But there are only certain paths through this wall. These transporters need a high concentration of creatine in the blood for them to transport creatine into muscle. This transport is also controlled by the creatine content of muscle, with there being a clear upper limit to muscle creatine concentration. Indeed, for those who don't see an increase in muscle creatine content with creatine supplementation, one of the likely reasons is that their muscle creatine content is at the known limit. In contrast, vegetarians have a low dietary intake of creatine, leading to a low muscle creatine content. In this group uptake into muscle is quicker and more effective. Most of us lie somewhere in the middle ground.

There are other ways to increase the speed of transport of creatine into muscle. The first is simply exercise. As is seen many times with many different transporters, in the post-exercise period the transport of creatine into muscle is more effective than at rest. As such it is clear that the timing of creatine supplementation plays a role in maximizing uptake into muscle, with the post-exercise period being the most effective time.

The second way to increase creatine transport into the muscle is to consume enough carbohydrate to increase the storage hormone insulin. Insulin interacts with the creatine transporter on the muscle cell wall to increase transport, and increases in response to intake of carbohydrates and some proteins. Therefore, consuming creatine with approximately 50g of carbohydrate seems to maximize creatine uptake into the muscle.

USING NUTRITION TO MAXIMIZE ADAPTATION TO STRENGTH TRAINING

> **RESEARCH FOCUS**
>
> **Timing of creatine and effects on muscle mass and strength gains (Antonio and Ciccone, 2013)**
>
> In 2013 research into the timing of creatine supplementation and the effects on resistance training adaptations was conducted. Nineteen male bodybuilders were recruited, and were allocated to two different experimental groups. The first group consumed 5g of creatine immediately before resistance exercise. The second group consumed this immediately after training. The participants trained for five days per week for five weeks.
>
> The group that supplemented creatine after exercise appeared to get bigger gains from the training. The post-training group increased their muscle mass by an average of 1.8kg over four weeks, whereas the pre-training group only increased muscle mass by 0.9kg over the same time period. The post-training group increased their one repetition maximum bench press by an average of 8.2kg (8.8 in diagram), compared to 6.6kg in the pre group.
>
> | | Change in muscle mass (kg) | Change in 1 RM Bench Press (kg) |
> |---|---|---|
> | Pre-Exercise Creatine | 0.8 | 6.6 |
> | Post-Exercise Creatine | 1.8 | 8.8 |
>
> *Changes in muscle mass and bench press performance during a four-week training period supplementing creatine before or after training.*
>
> Consuming creatine post-exercise is more effective than consuming it pre-exercise. This is primarily because creatine is more readily taken up into the muscle after exercise.

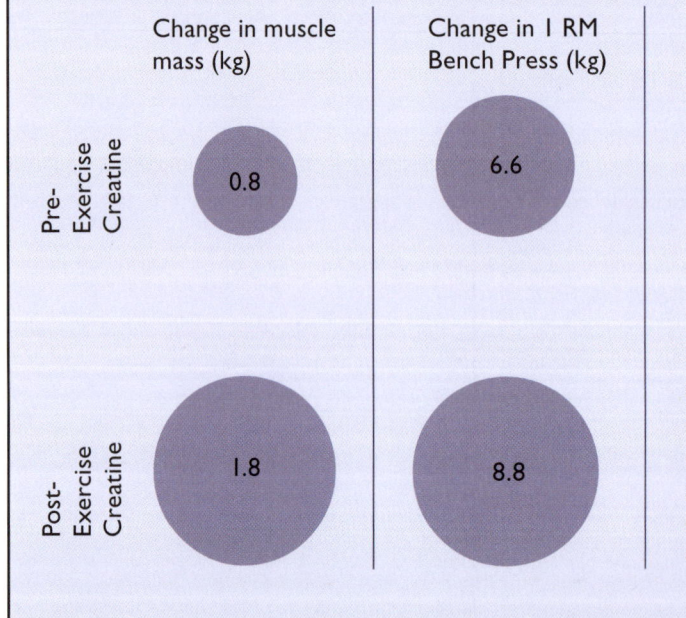

Once in the muscle, creatine is stored with water. The athlete will therefore see an increase in body weight of up to 1kg just by an increase in water storage within the muscle. This increase in water storage can have an effect by itself by increasing cell swelling. This cell swelling effect acts as a stressor on the muscle and leads to muscle growth.

A one-off dose of creatine is not effective, though. To elevate muscle creatine content and allow this elevation to continue, creatine needs to be taken over a longer period of

USING NUTRITION TO MAXIMIZE ADAPTATION TO STRENGTH TRAINING

time. The most traditional way to increase muscle creatine content is to 'load' with 20g per day for five to seven days and then follow this up with a 'maintenance' dose of 3–5g for two to three weeks, followed by a rest week and then repeat. This approach appears to have entered the dogma of practice across many athletes. However, it may not be necessary. Many of the original studies looking into creatine took this approach, and it does indeed lead to an increased muscle creatine content, but so does a daily dose of 3–5g over the same time period. The increase in muscle creatine content may not be as quick, but it will get to the same end point.

The loading and then maintenance approach to creatine supplementation is a good example of how research can be 'photocopied' and then enter dogma. The studies that began with a loading dose followed by maintenance were looking at timeframes for an increase in creatine and then its subsequent decline, and if the increased muscle creatine content could be maintained with a smaller dose. They were not designed to provide an optimal dosing protocol, but were effective in answering the questions the researchers were looking at.

So you've taken your 5g of creatine per day, and your muscle creatine content has increased. Will it make your fingers click and keep clicking? Well, it won't affect the first click, but will affect the second and the third and so on. The evidence is clear that when performing exercise of 2–30s in duration on a repeated basis with rest periods of 30s to five minutes, performance will be improved.

This ability to perform high-intensity exercise repeatedly has relevance for strength training adaptation. Creatine by itself might not make you stronger or bigger, although the jury is out on this one. What it will almost certainly do is allow you to train harder when you do train. By pushing out one more set at a slightly higher intensity over time, these effects will build to a greater strength gain than if creatine wasn't supplemented. It is this interaction between resistance exercise and creatine which is key and can be used as a training aid to maximize strength gains from a strength training programme.

CREATINE AND HEALTH

Over the years there have been lots of questions asked with regard to creatine and health outcomes. To date there has been no evidence of any side effects in what amounts to over 1,000 scientific publications on creatine, and it is one of the world's most used supplements.

It seems that creatine has other uses in muscle building. A Cochrane review, one of the highest levels of evidence in science, has shown that there is emerging evidence of creatine playing a role in improving muscle strength and functional performance in muscular dystrophies.

Alongside this, there is evidence that creatine supplementation may delay the loss of muscle mass and muscle strength that comes with ageing, as well as having a role in maintaining brain function in old age. It will be interesting to see the development of these areas in the coming years.

Other supplements

Creatine may be the king of supplements when it comes to building muscle strength and mass, but there are certainly many more on the market, with wonderful claims about their use and the results you will get from taking them. Three other supplements are worth considering.

USING NUTRITION TO MAXIMIZE ADAPTATION TO STRENGTH TRAINING

Supplement Cons

- Risk of inadvertent coping
- Risk to health
- Limited scientific evidence for most products.

Ask yourself:

- What is the evidence for the product?
- Can I get it from my diet?
- Does it sound too good to be true?
- Am I just looking for a magic bullet?

- Simple and pragmatic to use
- Some such as creatine and beta-alanine have good evidence to support their use

Supplement Pros

Pros and cons of nutritional supplements.

Beta-alanine is one such supplement. The mechanisms behind its function are discussed in detail in Chapter 8. However, in summary beta-alanine is one of the precursors, and the rate-limiting precursor, of the intramuscular buffer carnosine. Supplementation is over a chronic time period, with daily ingestion of up to 5g per day shown to increase muscle carnosine content. While there appear to be no direct effects on muscle strength and power in events that last less than 60s, there is some evidence that beta-alanine supplementation can lead to a greater training performance, and subsequently increase the adaptation from strength training. It also appears that beta-alanine can improve the effect of creatine in enhancing training performance.

β-hydroxy β-methylbutyrate, or HMB as it is more commonly known, is marketed as a supplement that can help support muscle growth and strength gains. HMB is a metabolite of the amino acid leucine, which as we will see in the following section is essential for muscle growth. HMB in clinical situations appears to be effective in preventing muscle breakdown. However, this has not been shown in athlete populations to a conclusive degree. In situations where muscle breakdown needs to be reduced, 1–3g of HMB daily may be of use.

More recently, interest in the phospholipid phosphatidic acid (PA) has shown promising results in increasing muscle mass and strength. Muscle contraction leads to an

USING NUTRITION TO MAXIMIZE ADAPTATION TO STRENGTH TRAINING

increase in cell concentration of PA. Subsequent to this increase, PA interacts with the mammalian target of rapamyacin (mTOR). mTOR appears to be the molecular regulator of muscle growth. The interaction of PA and mTOR leads to stimulation of muscle growth. A handful of papers have now shown that supplementation with PA can lead to an increase in both muscle strength and size when supplemented at a rate of approximately 750mg per day. However, these studies have been conducted in less than optimal dietary conditions for muscle growth, in particular in conditions of low leucine diets. Despite this, it is a promising supplement for muscle growth.

Other areas to consider are acute manipulations prior to training sessions, which will lead to an increase in strength training performance and subsequently to greater strength gains. In particular, caffeine could be a potent performance enhancer. There is increasing evidence that intake of 1–3mg per kg of caffeine thirty to sixty minutes prior to a resistance exercise session will lead to greater performance in the session. Ultimately this will hopefully lead to greater increases in strength gains in the long term.

There are a number of supplements that could be discussed here. However, at present there is little evidence for using any other supplement apart from the ones discussed

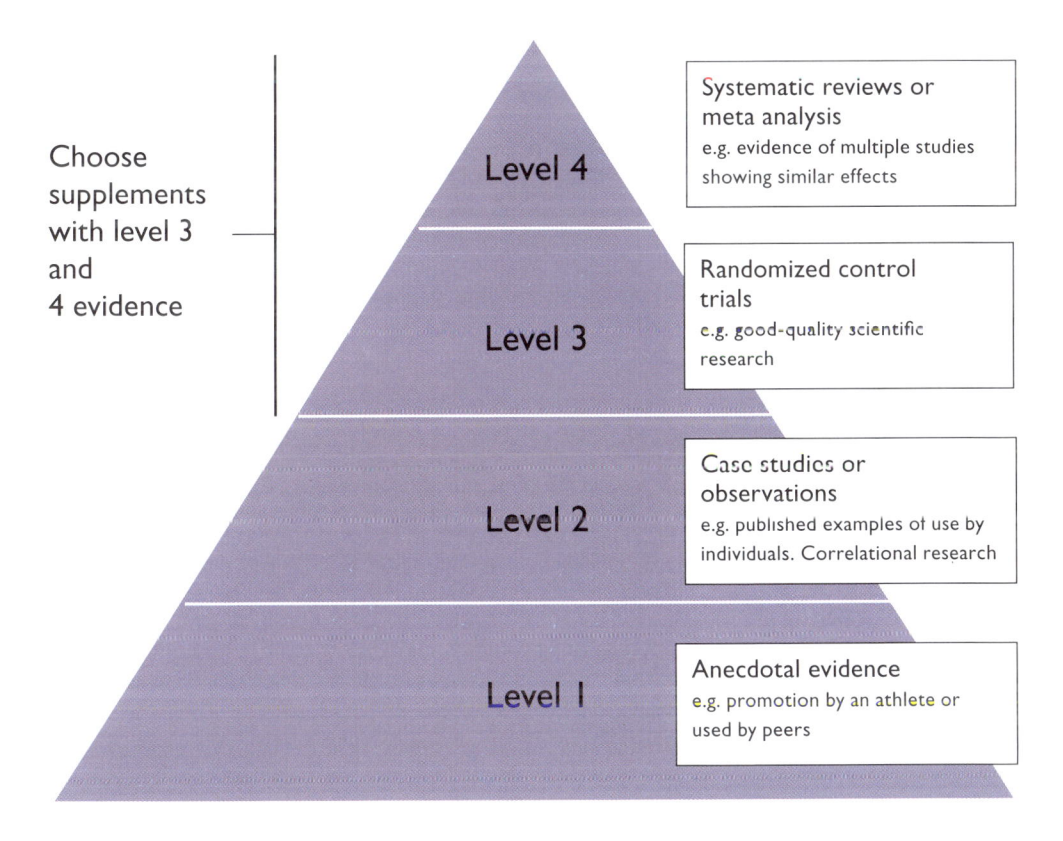

Choose supplements with level 3 and 4 evidence

Level 4 — Systematic reviews or meta analysis
e.g. evidence of multiple studies showing similar effects

Level 3 — Randomized control trials
e.g. good-quality scientific research

Level 2 — Case studies or observations
e.g. published examples of use by individuals. Correlational research

Level 1 — Anecdotal evidence
e.g. promotion by an athlete or used by peers

Levels of evidence for supplements.

USING NUTRITION TO MAXIMIZE ADAPTATION TO STRENGTH TRAINING

above. So don't be conned by the marketing hype. There are a handful that will help; other than that, don't waste your money.

Protein

So if you want to get massive and grow more muscle to get stronger you need lots of hormones, right? Post-exercise you need to increase hormones as much as possible to maximize the adaptation? Well, maybe not so much. Over the last few years the evidence seems to point to the fact that you can increase muscle hypertrophy in the absence of post-exercise hormonal increases.

Despite this, the main hormones that have been investigated in terms of post-exercise skeletal hypertrophy have been insulin-like growth factor I (IGF-I), growth hormone (GH) and testosterone. The evidence seems reasonably clear that IGF-I and GH have minimal effect on muscle growth.

What about testosterone, though? That's the one all the dopers use to get massive, isn't it? Indeed it is and research is clear that if you take super-physiological doses of testosterone then you will gain significant amounts of muscle and strength. In a classic study from 2001 Shalender Bhasin and colleagues showed that muscle strength and size increased in a dose-dependent manner with increased doses of testosterone administration. So it seems that more is better in terms of testosterone. However, taking this approach will violate the World Anti-Doping Code and lead to an anti-doping violation.

Can nutrition do anything to 'boost' testosterone to this extent? The simple answer is no. Despite what supplement companies like to suggest and sell, there is no known legal supplement or diet that will 'boost' testosterone to the extent of making a difference to strength and muscle mass development. Those that have shown something only show changes that are within the daily variation of testosterone anyway. Essentially, taking a testosterone 'boosting' supplement is a bit like trying to find a needle in a haystack, and it's fair to say that it's a waste of money.

On the flip side, when testosterone production is inhibited in the human body there is a blunting of muscle growth and strength development. This could have significance for the diet of an athlete who is trying to gain muscle mass. A chronic period of time with low energy intake leads to a decrease in testosterone production. This chronic period of under-fuelling will cause a reduction in the ability of the body to hypertrophy and gain muscle mass.

There is also evidence that having a low fat or protein intake can affect testosterone production, although the evidence is not too strong. There is some evidence of a positive relationship between fat intake and both testosterone and oestrogen production in males and females respectively. Although fat in particular is under-researched, it has become common for fat intake to be decreased and demonized over the last five decades. Low fat intake could lead to an inability to produce testosterone. An athlete looking to gain mass should aim for 1.5g/kg of body weight per day to provide the stimulus for an appropriate hormonal environment.

Having adequate energy will lead to an anabolic environment in which the body can build muscle. In fact adequate energy is not only what is needed; it is likely that an increase in calorie intake is also necessary to increase muscle mass. As a general rule of thumb, to increase muscle mass an athlete should increase calorie intake by 500 kcal per day above the need to produce energy balance.

USING NUTRITION TO MAXIMIZE ADAPTATION TO STRENGTH TRAINING

Without doubt, the nutrient that has received the most attention in terms of muscle growth is protein. In fact you could think that's all you need to build bigger muscles, although that is not the case. So how important is it? If we start with a look at the desired outcomes of increased muscle strength and size, evidence seems to suggest that protein supplementation has a positive effect on both. Naomi Čermak, from the research group of Luc van Loon, undertook a systematic review of all studies that looked at the effect of protein supplementation on both strength and muscle size. The review showed that over an average of six weeks across twenty-two studies and with a total of 680 subjects undertaking resistance-type exercise, supplementing the diet with protein led to an average 0.69kg increase in muscle mass compared to a placebo. Using one repetition maximum (IRM) as a marker of strength gains, those who supplemented with protein on average had a 13.5kg greater increase in IRM compared to a placebo. This would seem to suggest that protein supplementation is important to increase both strength and size.

Turnover of skeletal muscle is a process that is in constant flux, and it is influenced by both exercise and dietary intake, particularly protein. When you eat or drink a source of protein, such as meat or milk, the protein is first digested in the stomach and then absorbed into the bloodstream through the small intestine in its constituent form of amino acids. There are around 500 known amino acids, but only twenty-three of them play a part in the building of proteins. These amino acids form together into chains, or polymers, to form proteins, which will then go on to have a particular function within the body. This could include formation of muscle cells and fibres, or formation of enzymes to produce energy within the body, or more structural aspects such as parts of the skin or eye.

Table 3.1 Essential and non-essential amino acids.

Essential Amino Acids	Non-essential Amino Acids
Histidine	Alanine
Isoleucine	Arginine
Leucine	Aspartic acid
Lysine	Cysteine
Methionine	Glutamic acid
Phenylalanine	Glutamine
Threonine	Glycine
Tryptophan	Proline
Valine	Serine
	Tyrosine
	Asparagine
	Selenocysteine

USING NUTRITION TO MAXIMIZE ADAPTATION TO STRENGTH TRAINING

Once digested, these amino acids travel through the blood to their site of action. In terms of our interest in growing muscles, we will focus on this as their end point. One of the amino acids stands out over the rest when it comes to skeletal muscle – this is the essential amino acid leucine. Leucine is the trigger that stimulates muscle growth at a molecular level by interacting with the molecular trigger of muscle growth, the mammalian target of rapamyacin (mTOR).

The leucine trigger hypothesis has developed out of the laboratory of Professor Stuart Phillips from McMaster University in Canada. Through a series of robust and elegant studies Professor Phillips' research group has shown that feeding high-leucine-containing proteins stimulates muscle protein synthesis once adequate leucine has been consumed. It has also shown that the 'threshold' for stimulation of protein synthesis is lowered with exercise, and increased with age, inactivity and disease.

When looking to choose a protein source to maximize muscle growth, whey protein seems to provide the optimal stimulus. Whey protein has been shown to provide a greater stimulus to muscle growth than soy protein, which in turn stimulates muscle growth to a greater extent than casein protein. These are good examples of what happens with protein ingestion. Whey protein has the highest leucine content compared to both casein and soy, and is absorbed quickly. This leads to a speedier appearance of leucine within the blood, resulting in a greater increase in muscle protein synthesis. However, it is not all about leucine content, as casein has a higher leucine content than soy but is digested significantly more slowly, leading to a slower appearance of leucine in the blood.

If it's all about leucine, then maybe only leucine should be used, or even just the essential amino acids? However, while this does provide an increase in leucine appearance in the blood similar to whey, and in the short term stimulates muscle protein synthesis, the effect appears to be for a shorter period of time. Therefore, it seems that whole proteins, particularly whey protein, provide the optimal source of protein to build muscle.

However, you can't survive on protein powders. So does the food you eat have the same effect? It appears so. Evidence so far has shown that both beef and milk will stimulate muscle protein synthesis, and in the case of milk it is more potent than soy at doing so.

Consuming protein and exercising have an independent and additive effect on muscle protein synthesis. If you consume a source of protein only, muscle protein synthesis will increase; similarly if you go to the gym and lift some weights, the same will happen. However, if you combine the two the magic really starts to happen and there is a significantly greater and more prolonged increase in muscle protein synthesis with the combination of resistance exercise and protein ingestion. Indeed, if the exercise stimulus is great enough then resistance exercise sensitizes the muscle to amino acids for up to twenty-four hours and potentially up to forty-eight hours after the exercise bout. Indeed, the appearance of amino acid transporters at the cell membrane of muscle is increased for at least twenty-four hours after an appropriate bout of exercise, which explains the increased sensitivity to amino acids after resistance exercise. Think of it as the muscle opening more doors after exercise to allow the amino acids to enter the muscle.

So if taking part in resistance training can lead to an increase in sensitivity of muscle to amino acids for up to forty-eight hours, timing is important. We have been conditioned to think that post-exercise protein intake is essential to maximize recovery and adapta-

USING NUTRITION TO MAXIMIZE ADAPTATION TO STRENGTH TRAINING

tion to exercise. However, this may not be the case. When timing is investigated in longitudinal studies there seems to be very little effect on muscle mass gains or strength. However, focusing timing of protein immediately after exercise may confer one benefit as it is a simple way to increase total protein intake. In order to maximize hypertrophy gains, an increased protein intake is needed. Getting an athlete to consume protein immediately post-exercise is a pragmatic way to increase total protein intake. There are also other benefits to timing nutrient intake post-exercise, such as consuming carbohydrate to maximize muscle glycogen resynthesis and to support the immune system.

While timing post-exercise does not appear to be as important as first thought, it is also not advisable for athletes to consume all their protein in one sitting. In order to maximize muscle protein synthesis a recent series of studies has shown that spreading the daily dose of protein intake into four to eight meals per day is more beneficial than consuming the same total amount of protein in one or two sittings. When you look at a normal dietary pattern for athletes or non-athletes, a large intake of protein in one sitting is common. It is common for breakfast to have minimal protein, lunch potentially the same, and to have a large protein intake in the evening, with snacks often having limited protein content. It is advisable for athletes to spread out their protein intake throughout the day to maximize the muscle protein synthesis response to exercise. This will also help support appetite regulation, as protein is the most filling of all nutrients.

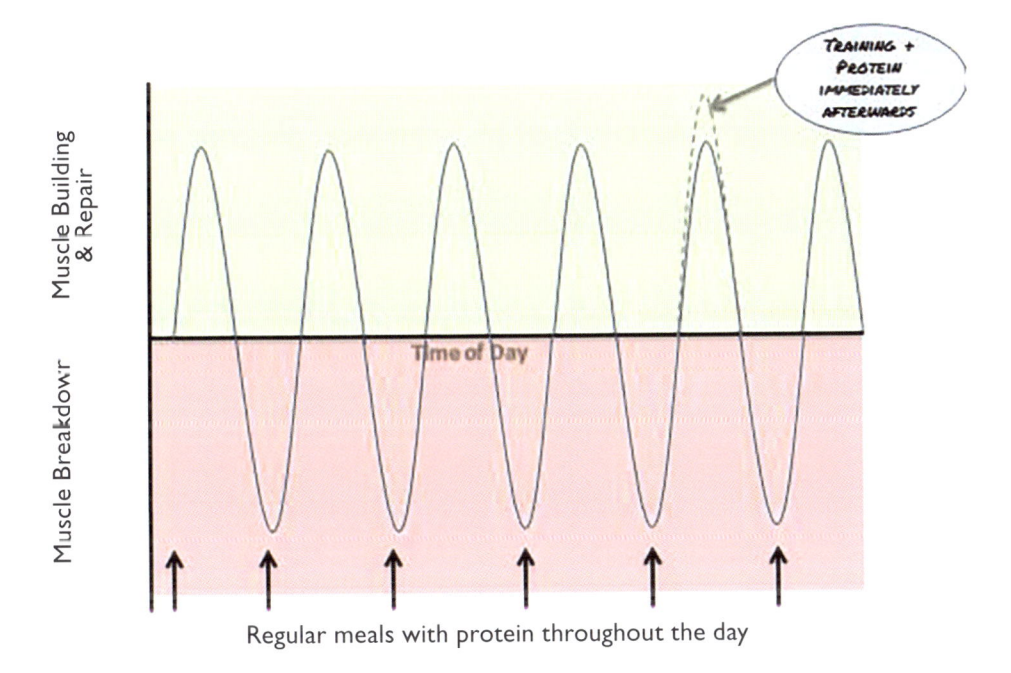

Optimal intake of protein during a day to maximize muscle building and repair. As can be seen, protein interacts with exercise to lead to a greater anabolic response. Black arrows indicate intake of protein.

43

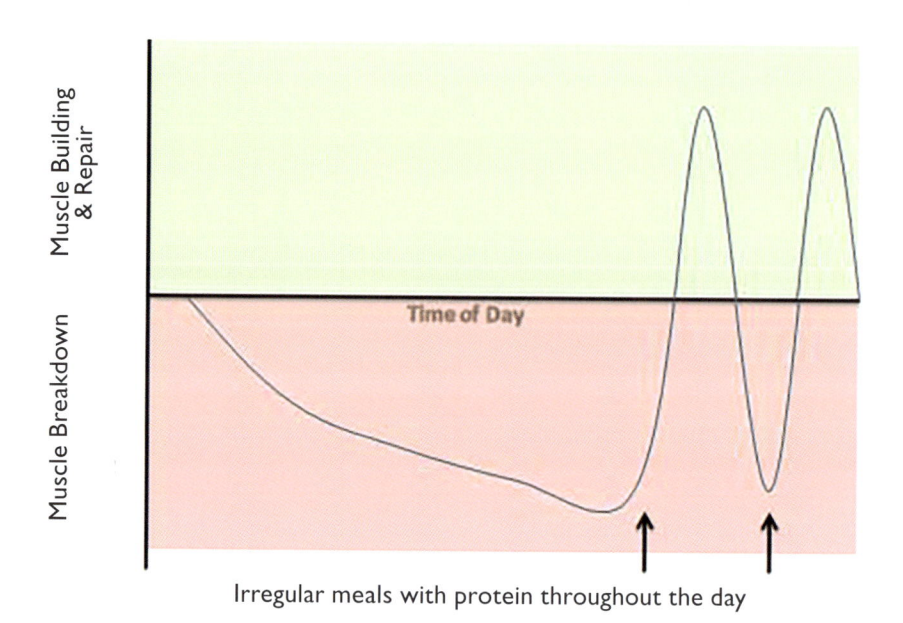

USING NUTRITION TO MAXIMIZE ADAPTATION TO STRENGTH TRAINING

Irregular meals with protein throughout the day

Sub-optimal distribution of protein intake in a day, yet this is typical of many diets. As can be seen, this leads to a high proportion of time spent where the muscle is in a catabolic state. Black arrows indicate intake of protein.

The reason for taking smaller doses of protein on a regular basis can be seen in the dose response relationship between protein intake and muscle protein synthesis. Again, a series of studies from the laboratory of Professor Stuart Phillips at McMaster University has shown that ingestion of only 10g of protein can stimulate muscle protein synthesis, with 20g providing an even greater stimulation. However, 40g does not seem to confer a significantly greater effect. The extra protein seems to be used for energy, rather than muscle building. If this is taken relative to body weight, the relationship appears to suggest that muscle protein synthesis can be maximally stimulated at around 0.3 g/kg of body weight per meal.

There are two caveats to this 0.3g/kg of body weight per meal. The first is that immediately pre-bed a greater dose may be needed. It appears that a protein dose of approximately 0.6g/kg of body weight before sleep leads to an increase in muscle protein synthesis while sleeping. Given athletes should look to sleep for at least eight hours, this is a good opportunity to ensure the body continues to build muscle during a key period of recovery.

The second caveat is a need for greater protein intake in the older athlete. With ageing, and particularly above the age of fifty, a process called anabolic resistance begins to set in. This makes the muscle less sensitive to protein intake. Therefore, in older athletes a protein dose of around 0.4g per kg of body

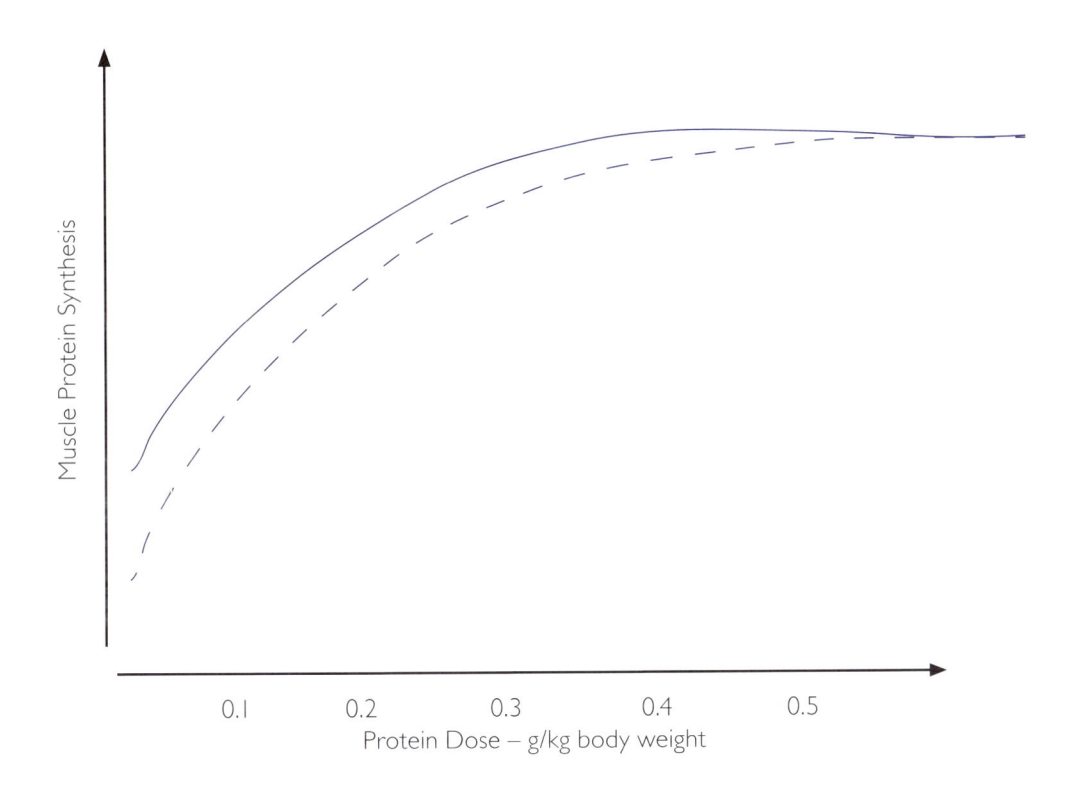

USING NUTRITION TO MAXIMIZE ADAPTATION TO STRENGTH TRAINING

Dose/response curve for protein intake and muscle protein synthesis. Solid line is the response of whey protein; dotted line indicates shift in dose/response curve with other proteins such as soy, and also how inactivity affects the dose response curve of protein.

weight is recommended to maximize muscle protein synthesis.

In practical terms to maximize muscle protein synthesis, and therefore muscle mass gains and strength gains, an athlete should look to have four portions of protein in a day: 0.3g/kg of body weight of protein per meal, with a portion of protein prior to bed of around 0.6g/kg of body weight per day.

What about other nutrients taken post-exercise to maximize muscle protein synthesis? It was originally thought that carbohydrate ingestion was essential to maximize this. However, it has since been shown that this is not the case, and muscle protein synthesis can occur in the absence of carbohydrate intake. Taking this finding in isolation may lead one to conclude that carbohydrate is not needed in the post-exercise feed after resistance training. Resistance training is fuelled by muscle glycogen, though, and a failure to restore this with carbohydrate intake may lead to a decreased performance in subsequent exercise sessions. There is also an increased stress on the body whenever

USING NUTRITION TO MAXIMIZE ADAPTATION TO STRENGTH TRAINING

Table 3.2 **20g sources of protein.**

Food	Weight	Handy Measure
Beef, lamb, pork	75g	2 medium slices
Turkey, chicken	75g	1 small breast
Liver	100g	2 tablespoons
Grilled fish	100g	1 small fillet
Salmon/tuna	100g	1 small tin
Sardines	100g	1 small tin
Shrimps/prawns	100g	2 tablespoons
Eggs	–	3 medium
Cheddar cheese	75g	2 matchbox size pieces
Cottage cheese	150g	4 tablespoons
Milk – skimmed/semi-skimmed	600ml	1 pint
Greek yogurt	150g	4 tablespoons

ALCOHOL AND MUSCLE GROWTH

It's Friday evening, and you've just been to the gym. You've drunk 20g of whey protein, mixed with 50g of carbohydrate. You've maximized muscle protein synthesis with the whey protein, and recovery with the carbohydrate. You meet your friends in the pub on the way home. One beer leads to two, to three, and before you know it you're waking up with a hangover. Meanwhile, your body is working to undo all the hard work you did in the gym the night before, lifting those weights, drinking the protein shake and recovering with carbohydrates. That's because alcohol intake has been shown to inhibit muscle protein synthesis significantly. So if you want to get big, hold back on the beer.

muscle glycogen concentration is decreased, leading to a greater risk of injury and illness. There are likely to be other benefits to consuming carbohydrate along with protein in the post-exercise period.

Summary

- Nutrition acts as a facilitator for training adaptation. The appropriate training stimulus is key to providing the desired training

USING NUTRITION TO MAXIMIZE ADAPTATION TO STRENGTH TRAINING

effect. However, appropriate timing and type of nutrition added around training can lead to a greater training effect than if appropriate nutrition was not present.

- One of the most common adaptations to resistance training is hypertrophy. This is due to the relationship between the cross-sectional area of a muscle and the ability of the muscle to produce force.
- Protein intake appears to be the greatest stimulator for facilitating hypertrophy adaptation. Skeletal muscle is in constant flux where it is being formed and broken down consistently. The aim of hypertrophy training is to shift protein balance in favour of muscle formation. Protein allows this to happen.
- The amino acid leucine appears to play a key role in triggering muscle growth. It acts as the molecular trigger for muscle growth as seen in the leucine trigger hypothesis. However, without other amino acids found in whole proteins muscle growth will not be as effective.
- Alcohol intake may lead to a decrease in muscle mass gains during resistance exercise.

Gold

Creatine: Creatine is a peptide naturally formed within the body, and allows the muscle to perform high-intensity contractions. Supplementing with creatine monohydrate at a dose of 3–5g per day for thirty days will significantly increase creatine stores within the muscle. This should be timed after exercise to maximize creatine uptake into the muscle. Consuming creatine with a source of carbohydrate will also allow for greater gains in muscle uptake. Supplementation has been shown to increase the amount of work that can be produced during resistance exercise, therefore increasing strength gains in the long term.

Protein intake: Total protein intake does appear to be important in the increase of muscle mass in particular. Aiming for 2–3g of protein per kg of body weight per day will help facilitate muscle mass gains.

Silver

Carbohydrate feeding pre- and post-training: Muscle glycogen provides a significant source of energy for resistance-type exercise. Including some sort of carbohydrate in the pre-training meal will allow for greater training performance. Consume approximately 1g per kg of body weight prior to a workout, and a similar amount after training. Prioritize timing around training over consuming carbohydrates at other times of the day to fit these into your overall daily carbohydrate needs.

Protein partitioning: Maximal protein synthesis occurs after ingestion of 0.3g of protein per kg of body weight. This therefore promotes the need to consume four to six meals containing this amount of protein per day to allow total protein needs to be maintained.

Protein type: Whey protein appears to be the most effective type of protein to promote gains in muscle protein synthesis. However, food sources such as beef and milk have been shown to be effective, too. Whey protein should be chosen in the post-exercise period to maximize absorption of leucine. However, food sources should be chosen in other situations as it is unrealistic to expect each meal to be based on supplementation and may lead to other nutrient deficiencies.

Caffeine: Intake of 1–3mg per kg of body weight thirty to sixty minutes prior to a resistance exercise session may help promote performance in the gym.

47

Bronze

Beta-alanine supplementation: Supplementation with 5g per day may allow a greater workload to occur during resistance exercise. It may work synergistically with creatine to increase training load.

HMB: 3g per day may reduce muscle breakdown, therefore leading to increases in muscle mass. More evidence is needed, though, to conclusively prove this.

Phosphatidic acid: 750mg per day may influence molecular pathways which promote muscle growth. However, limited evidence to suggest this works in synergy with protein.

Protein timing: There is minimal evidence that protein timing is essential for muscle growth. After resistance exercise the muscle is sensitized to protein intake for up to seventy-two hours. While it will do no harm, and may have other benefits such as muscle soreness management, it is not essential for muscle growth.

Further reading

Antonio, J. & Ciccone, V. (2013). The effects of pre-versus post-workout supplementation of creatine monohydrate on body composition and strength. *Journal of the International Society of Sports Nutrition*, 10(1), 36.

Table 3.3 Example diet plan for Chapter 3.

Meal	Food
Breakfast	Large bowl of porridge made with semi-skimmed milk, with walnuts and raspberries, topped with 125g of Greek yogurt 1 apple 1 probiotic yogurt Cup of coffee with 2 espresso shots
Post-exercise	20g of whey protein with 35g of carbohydrates 1 apple
Lunch	1 baked salmon fillet with a baked sweet potato and a mixed salad
Snack	2 slices of wholemeal bread with almond butter
Post-exercise	1 pint of semi-skimmed milk made into a smoothie with blueberries
Dinner	1 chicken breast with brown rice, broccoli, kale and carrots 1 avocado
Pre-bed snack	125g of Greek yogurt with chopped nuts and berries

Carbohydrate (g/kg body weight)	Protein (g/kg body weight)	Fat (g/kg body weight)
4.7	2.6	1.5

Cermak, N. M., Res, P. T., de Groot, L. C. P. G. M., Saris, W. H. M. & van Loon, L. J. C. (2012). Protein supplementation augments the adaptive response of skeletal muscle to resistance-type exercise training: a meta-analysis. *The American Journal of Clinical Nutrition*, 96(6), 1454–64.

McGlory, C. & Phillips, S. M. (2014). Assessing the regulation of skeletal muscle plasticity in response to protein ingestion and resistance exercise: recent developments. *Current Opinion in Clinical Nutrition and Metabolic Care*, 17(5), 412–7.

CHAPTER 4

CONCURRENT TRAINING AND BUFFER CAPACITY

Many sporting events are not purely based on endurance, nor on strength. They are a combination of the two. Athletes may find it difficult to find the time to train for the different components of their event. Sports such as rowing and track cycling need a combination of high-volume endurance training, interval training at around race pace and strength training. There may be a need to weave into the training week some sort of technical or tactical training, too.

Concurrent training

Food consumed around training can act as a facilitator to training adaptation, either amplifying or dampening the training effect depending on the desired response. In essence, for those who need to undertake concurrent training, nutrition can act as a way of shortcutting some of the training adaptations needed and provide a time-efficient way to get the most out of training.

The need to perform both strength training and aerobic training is a challenge, as they interact with each other to interfere with the adaptive response to training. Endurance training, in particular, seems to prevent the adaptation to strength training. This interference effect was first established by the seminal research of Robert Hickson in 1980, with work conducted at the University of Illinois at Chicago Circle. Hickson took three groups of untrained subjects and got them to perform three different types of exercise training for ten weeks. The first group performed thirty to forty minutes of strength training five times per week. The second group performed thirty to forty minutes per day of aerobic training five times per week. Finally, the third group performed both types of training five days per week for ten weeks.

The group that performed only aerobic training increased their VO_2 max, the marker of aerobic fitness, by 25 per cent. There was a similar magnitude of change in the group that performed both types of training. In the group that performed the strength only training there was no change in VO_2 max. So far, this is what Hickson expected to see: you perform aerobic training, and you adapt to it.

However, the strength training adaptations showed some interesting outcomes. Unsurprisingly, those who only performed aerobic training did not really improve their strength. In both the strength group and the strength and aerobic group there were gains in strength over the first seven weeks of training. However, beyond this time point the change in strength levelled out in the aerobic and strength group.

Interference of aerobic training on strength gains is an effect that has been consistently shown over the last thirty years since Hickson's research. Running-type exercise seems to inhibit muscle strength and growth to a greater extent than cycling. Similarly the greater the volume of aerobic training undertaken, the greater the inhibition of gains in muscle strength and hypertrophy.

The exact mechanism of how aerobic training interferes with gains in muscle strength and size has not been elucidated. However, one potential mechanism comes at a molecular level. The molecular trigger that leads to hypertrophy is the mammalian target of rapamyacin (mTOR). mTOR is inhibited by a by product of aerobic exercise AMPK, which is produced in response to an increase in the muscular concentration of AMP and calcium. At a molecular level this inhibition of mTOR by AMPK may explain some of the interference effect.

In order to understand the role of nutrition in maximizing both the aerobic and strength component of concurrent training, let's walk through two different training situations. The first will involve a long slow run of, say, ninety minutes, followed five hours later by a session in the gym. The second will involve a gym session followed by a sixty-minute bike ride.

So our athlete wakes and gets ready for the ninety-minute run. In order to maximize the aerobic adaptations to this exercise they are going to do this before breakfast, so they drink a quick coffee and off they go for a run. Ninety minutes later they return home. The signalling pathways in the muscle kick into action in response to the exercise. Those that trigger the signals to ultimately adapt to the exercise training begin. The master regulator of aerobic adaptations, PGC1-α, is upregulated to ultimately lead to an enhancement of aerobic enzymes and mitochondria. One of the stimulants for this process is an increase in the enzyme AMPK due to an increase in free calcium in the muscle and the metabolite AMP. Over the next three hours AMPK levels gradually return to resting levels.

So what should our athlete eat after the long, slow run? Protein is a given, as this will enhance post-exercise protein synthesis, primarily of the structural protein that makes up the muscle rather than the production of enzymes themselves. If the goal is to maintain muscle mass or even lead to growth of muscle, protein intake prior to exercise should also be considered as this will reduce the catabolic effect of running in particular and will not inhibit any aerobic adaptations to the training.

What about carbohydrate, though; will this inhibit any training adaptations? If taken before or during the run then quite possibly it will reduce the effectiveness of the long, slow run in terms of enhancing the aerobic adaptations to training. However, it is likely that it will have minimal effect on aerobic training adaptations post-exercise. Withholding carbohydrates post-exercise also increases the risk of illness.

Consuming a mixture of carbohydrates and protein will not inhibit adaptation to aerobic training, and may enhance it. It will almost certainly enhance the ability to perform in the second session of the day. Therefore our athlete consumes 20g of protein, equivalent to 0.3g/kg of body mass, which has been shown to be the optimum amount to enhance muscle protein synthesis – so, let's say a pint of milk. Alongside this the athlete consumes 70g of quickly absorbing carbohydrate; there are some carbohydrates in the milk already so we add in one large banana and an apple. Together with this the athlete consumes 1.5l of fluid in the time between finishing the run and starting the gym session to offset the fluids lost in the first training session. Of course, the milk contributes to the fluid intake, too. Approximately two

CONCURRENT TRAINING AND BUFFER CAPACITY

hours before the start of the gym session the athlete consumes a chicken breast with a fist-size portion of rice and some vegetables as a meal, and is therefore ready to begin the gym session in an energy-replete state.

Before heading to the gym our athlete has a quick espresso coffee to get their approximate 100mg of caffeine. This will maximize their performance in the gym. They finish at the gym and want to maximize the adaptation to the training. They should look to consume 0.3g/kg of body weight of protein, preferably whey protein to maximize muscle protein synthesis, then two or three hours later consume a mixed meal, ensuring it contains a further 0.3g/kg of body weight of high leucine-containing protein, such as meat or fish. Then prior to bed they should consume 0.4g/kg of slow-releasing protein such as casein to enhance muscle protein synthesis overnight.

Following this type of nutrition plan will maximize the adaptation to both training sessions while reducing the impact of the long, slow run on the second training session of the day. However, what if they are completed the other way around, the strength session first and the aerobic session second? Here things get a little more complicated, and the first question that needs to be asked is which is the greater adaptive need? If it is aerobic adaptations there will need to be consequences on strength gains; if it is strength gains there will need to be consequences for aerobic adaptations.

The main difference in terms of nutritional intervention comes in the second session. The first should be treated the same as any other gym-based workout that is aimed at increasing strength and muscle mass, as outlined in Chapter 3. However, the second aerobic session is where the nutritional intervention will differ. If the aim is to maximize aerobic adaptations then no carbohydrate should be consumed after the resistance exercise, during the aerobic session or even afterwards for one or two hours. This will, however, lead to a greater inhibition of strength gains.

This inhibition of strength gains is due to the increase in AMPK during the aerobic training session. The increase in AMPK inhibits mTOR, our regulator of muscle mass growth. mTOR is stimulated for up to seventy-two hours after a resistance exercise session, but will be switched off by AMPK increases due to the sixty-minute cycle ride. However, if we want to maximize the strength gains we should look to consume carbohydrate after the gym session, during the cycle and immediately after the cycle – for example, something like 50g of carbohydrate in a recovery shake post-gym session, 500ml of carbohydrate electrolyte drink during the cycle ride, and a pint of milk with a banana after the ride. This will lead to a smaller increase in AMPK, and subsequently less inhibition of mTOR.

These known interactions and interferences between training could be used deliberately to limit adaptations, in particular hypertrophy. Deliberately performing aerobic exercise after strength exercise, with minimal carbohydrate intake, will lead to a dampening of the hypertrophy response. In many sports, increasing strength without necessarily increasing mass is important. This could be one way to minimize mass gains.

Maximizing gains from interval training

Another key component of sports that require concurrent training is interval training. As these events are generally performed at or around VO_2 max, it is necessary to complete training sessions at intensities around this. Adaptations from this type of training are generally driven by the time spent at a given intensity. The aim is to use a variety of work-

CONCURRENT TRAINING AND BUFFER CAPACITY

to-rest ratios to spend as much time as possible at the given intensity. Generally this is at a high intensity.

Carbohydrate

For the body to produce energy at these high intensities it is important that hydrogen ions are produced, which are primarily a function of the use of glycolysis to produce ATP. Glycolysis is the breakdown of carbohydrates to produce energy. In order for the body to work effectively at high intensities muscle glycogen needs to be present within the muscle at adequate concentrations, therefore enabling exercise to take place at sufficient intensity. It is clear from research regarding exercising in a glycogen-depleted state that exercise intensity is reduced during interval training, and subsequently there is a reduction in the adaptations to glycolytic pathways and enzymes with low carbohydrate intake. When it comes to interval training, carbohydrate is king.

We can start to see the effects of diet and interval training at a biochemical level. Pyruvate dehydrogenase (PDH) is a rate-limiting enzyme in the conversion of pyruvate, which is the end point of glycolysis, to acetyl coA and therefore entry into the mitochondria for further oxidation and energy production. A key adaptation to interval training is an increase in activity of PDH, both at rest and during exercise.

There are also links between increased PDH and high-intensity exercise performance. Indeed, one of the reasons a high-

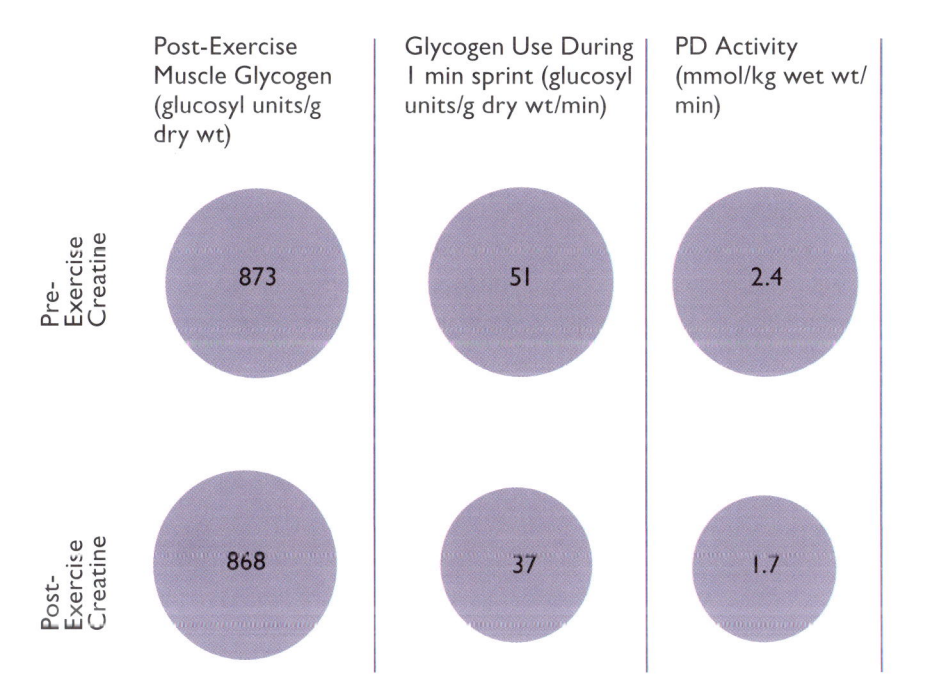

	Post-Exercise Muscle Glycogen (glucosyl units/g dry wt)	Glycogen Use During 1 min sprint (glucosyl units/g dry wt/min)	PD Activity (mmol/kg wet wt/min)
Pre-Exercise Creatine	873	51	2.4
Post-Exercise Creatine	868	37	1.7

Changes in glycogen storage, glycogen use and enzyme activity during sprint exercise following a high-fat or high-carbohydrate diet. Following a high-fat diet there is an inhibition of the muscles' ability to use carbohydrate as a fuel and therefore produce high power outputs. (Adapted from Stellingwerff et al., 2006.)

intensity warm-up is an effective way to improve potential prior to high-intensity performance is the increases in PDH activity seen after the warm-up.

However, what we eat has an effect on PDH. A high-fat diet will decrease resting PDH and any increases in PDH during exercise, and blunt the adaptation seen during exercise training. Conversely a high-carbohydrate diet will increase PDH both at rest and during exercise. Therefore, it is important that to maximize performance gains from interval training the training should be performed in a high-carbohydrate state. If it is performed in a low-carbohydrate state, there is a risk of inhibiting the adaptation to training.

Creatine

Beyond the daily diet of the athlete, there are a number of supplements that can enhance the adaptation to high-intensity interval training, one of which is creatine supplementation. As outlined in Chapter 3, the purpose of creatine supplementation is to increase the storage of phosphocreatine in the muscle cell itself. One consequence of increasing the muscle creatine content is that the recovery of this content after a short exercise bout is enhanced; perfect for interval training, where the aim is quite often to produce high amounts of intensity, then recover and go again.

So in theory, supplementing with creatine then performing high-intensity interval training should allow the athlete to spend more time at a higher intensity overall and therefore enhance the adaptation to training. Does the research support this? A series of studies from the University of Oklahoma, in the laboratory of Professor Jeff Stout, seems to suggest so.

In these series of research studies healthy, male, college-age students were split into three groups: a group that had no treatment, another that took a placebo, and a final group that supplemented with 10g of creatine per day. Following supplementation, the three different groups undertook a four-week high-intensity interval training programme.

The findings were interesting. Anaerobic work capacity is a marker of high-intensity exercise performance. No changes were seen in the variable. However, in some of the more aerobic markers of performance, such as critical power (the highest power output the athlete can sustain in a physiologic steady state), this and ventilatory threshold were increased. These are important markers for many endurance events.

Therefore, it appears that there is evidence that supplementing with creatine prior to high-intensity exercise training can enhance the adaptation to the training. Primarily this is by allowing the athlete to train harder for longer.

Caffeine

To increase performance in a given high-intensity interval training session and therefore increase time at a higher training intensity, caffeine is an effective ergogenic aid. Caffeine has consistently been shown in research to enhance performance across a variety of exercise intensities, including many which would be experienced when interval training.

An acute dose of 3mg/kg of body weight of caffeine, sixty minutes prior to an interval training session, will lead to an increase in performance within that session. Subsequent to this an increased adaptation will be seen.

Caffeine is also effective at increasing performance in interval training when the training is performed in a nutritionally inadequate state. The research group of Professor John Hawley in Australia took a group of athletes through four different trials. They performed eight five-minute interval sessions with either a high or a low muscle

CONCURRENT TRAINING AND BUFFER CAPACITY

glycogen state, with either 3mg/kg of body weight of caffeine or placebo taken one hour prior to the start of the interval training session.

Training with normal muscle glycogen concentrations was seen as the 'normal' state when placebo was also co-ingested. During this condition the participants had an average power output during the interval training of around 77 per cent of peak power output (PPO). When caffeine was taken prior to this the average peak power output during the interval training sessions was increased to nearly 80 per cent of PPO.

Training with low muscle glycogen and a placebo reduced the average power output during the training session to 71 per cent of PPO. Adding caffeine on top of this increased the average power to 74 per cent of PPO. Clearly, training in a low muscle glycogen state reduces the intensity of training, and while caffeine does attenuate this slightly, it can restore intensity to levels seen when training in a normal glycogen state. The study also shows that caffeine really can allow an athlete to train harder.

Carbohydrate intake during sessions

Consuming carbohydrate during training sessions would be a further way to maintain exercise intensity, leading to an overall greater workload than without the carbohydrate. During sessions that last for less than one hour in total duration the effect of carbohydrate is likely to be mediated by a stimulating effect on the brain, rather than a metabolic effect.

This stimulatory effect of carbohydrate has been shown quite nicely in studies looking at carbohydrate mouth-rinse and time-trial performance of up to one hour. From these studies it is clear that swilling carbohydrate around the mouth does lead to an increase in power output. There are receptors within the mouth that detect the presence of carbohydrate and send messages to the brain to that effect. These signals allow the brain to continue exercise in the belief that carbohydrate is on the way to support the metabolism.

For interval training mouth-swilling a carbohydrate gel in between intervals could be advantageous not only to increase

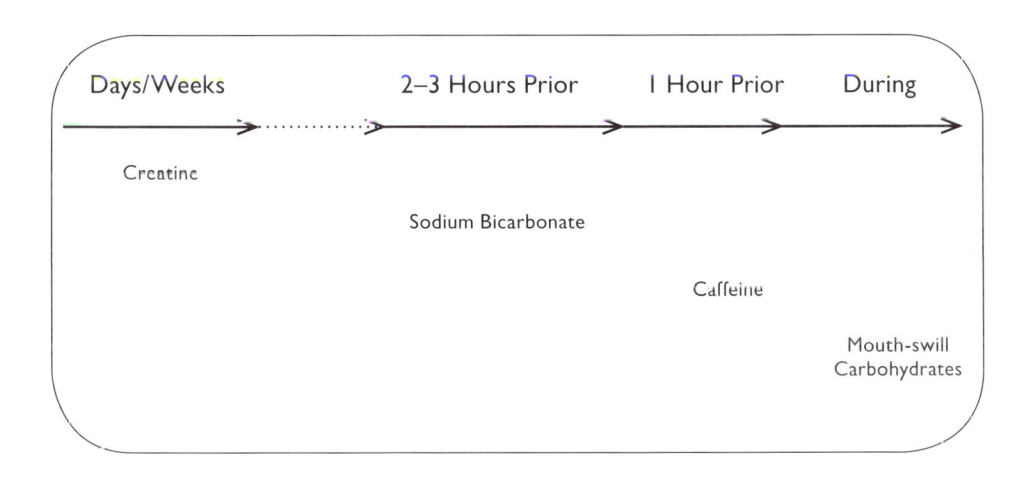

Timing of different interventions to influence adaptations to interval training.

CONCURRENT TRAINING AND BUFFER CAPACITY

exercise intensity, but to reduce any gastrointestinal distress that may occur as a consequence of swallowing a carbohydrate drink. Swilling carbohydrate around the mouth also seems to be most effective when the exercise is performed in a sub-optimal state, such as after a long period without food. This could be particularly important for busy athletes who have not had the opportunity to fuel optimally prior to a session.

Buffers

Along with interval training comes the inevitable production of acid, primarily from the production of energy through the glycolytic pathways. This is the stinging pain you feel when doing this type of exercise. Managing this acid production so that it does not reduce exercise intensity too much can be an effective way to support interval training.

Beta-alanine is a supplement that can help support the body's endogenous buffering system. It is the rate-limiting precursor of the dipeptide carnosine. Carnosine is one of the most important buffers of acid present within the muscle. Supplementing with 4–5g of beta-alanine per day for four to six weeks has been shown to increase the concentration of muscle carnosine, and subsequently increase exercise performance of events that last one to ten minutes in duration.

Generally intervals as part of training are one to ten minutes in duration and in principle this should mean that beta-alanine supplementation will support interval training performance. Research published in 2009 by Professor Jeff Stout suggests that this is the case. Healthy active males were placed on an interval training period for six weeks, either with or without beta-alanine (6g per day) supplementation. Those who were supplemented with beta-alanine showed a trend to performing more work at a higher intensity. This resulted in greater cardiorespiratory adaptations to the training period.

A further buffer that can be used to support interval training is sodium bicarbonate, more commonly known as baking soda. This ergogenic aid has been shown to effectively increase performance of events lasting between one and ten minutes – once again within the realm of interval training and potential improvements in performance.

Sodium bicarbonate works by increasing the bicarbonate concentration of the blood. This creates a gradient along which hydrogen ions (the main component causing an acidic environment within the muscle) can pass from the muscle into the blood, where they can be disposed of in the form of carbon dioxide.

Hydrogen ions, and in particular when bound to lactic acid in the form of lactate, pass from the muscle into the blood through monocarboxylic transporters, or MCT for short. An increase in these is seen through training anyway. However, when sodium bicarbonate is used prior to interval training sessions the number of MCTs found in the cell wall increases significantly. The outcome is a better ability to cope with high-intensity exercise – therefore magnifying the training effect.

Summary

- Many sporting events need a mixture of both endurance training and strength training. This can be very challenging to programme into a weekly plan. Many events also need the ability to perform high-intensity exercise, and with that a high capacity to cope with the acid produced by the muscles.
- The interaction between strength training and aerobic training is a challenge as they appear to interfere with each

CONCURRENT TRAINING AND BUFFER CAPACITY

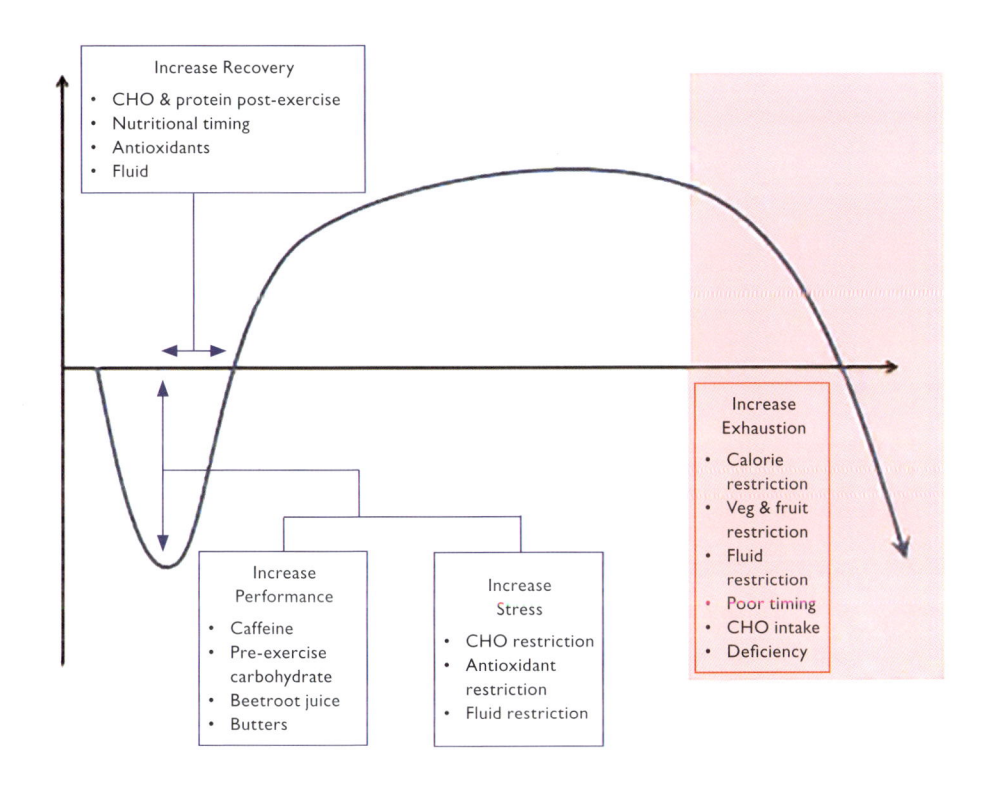

Increase Recovery
- CHO & protein post-exercise
- Nutritional timing
- Antioxidants
- Fluid

Increase Performance
- Caffeine
- Pre-exercise carbohydrate
- Beetroot juice
- Butters

Increase Stress
- CHO restriction
- Antioxidant restriction
- Fluid restriction

Increase Exhaustion
- Calorie restriction
- Veg & fruit restriction
- Fluid restriction
- Poor timing
- CHO intake
- Deficiency

How nutrition can influence training adaptation.

other's training adaptations. In particular there is evidence that endurance training can inhibit the long-term adaptations to strength training. This is termed 'concurrent training'. Appropriate food intake and timing can help minimize this interference effect.
- The influence of food and nutrients on the adaptations to concurrent training are primarily at the level of the molecular responses to training. However, this is only one potential mechanism by which aerobic training inhibits strength training.
- Interval training is a common training mode to increase performance at high intensities. Almost all interval training is performed at intensities that rely on carbohydrate as the predominant fuel source. Reductions in muscle glycogen concentration will lead to a reduction in performance in high-intensity exercise intervals.

Gold

Carbohydrate intake post-aerobic sessions: Consuming 1g of carbohydrate per kg of body weight will maximize resynthesis of muscle glycogen and minimize any molecular perturbations that may interfere with strength training.

Caffeine pre-sessions: Intake of 1–3mg of caffeine per kg of body weight thirty to sixty minutes prior to a training session where

CONCURRENT TRAINING AND BUFFER CAPACITY

there is a desire to perform at high intensities will improve performance of that training session.

Carbohydrates pre-interval training: Consuming 1g of carbohydrate per kg of body weight, one to three hours prior to the start of an interval training session, will promote adaptations to that training session, as well as promoting optimal performance.

Carbohydrate intake during interval sessions: Consuming 30–60g per hour of interval training will help maintain performance in the interval sessions, therefore leading to greater training adaptations. Mouth-swilling the carbohydrates around the mouth for twenty seconds may provide a similar benefit to swallowing the carbohydrates.

Silver

Creatine: Supplementing with 3–5g of creatine for thirty days will increase the creatine content of the muscle. This can lead to greater performance in high-intensity intervals, in particular those that involve very high intensities being repeated over a number of repetitions.

Table 4.1 Example diet plan for Chapter 4.

Meal	Food
Breakfast	Large bowl of porridge made with semi-skimmed milk, with walnuts and raspberries, topped with 125g of Greek yogurt 1 apple 1 probiotic yogurt Cup of coffee with 2 espresso shots
During exercise – 1 hour interval training	1 isotonic carbohydrate gel and 750ml of 6% carbohydrate electrolyte drink
Post-exercise	20g of whey protein with 35g of carbohydrates 1 apple
Lunch	1 tin of tuna with a baked sweet potato and a mixed salad
Snack	2 slices of wholemeal bread with almond butter
Post-exercise	1 pint of semi-skimmed milk made into a smoothie with blueberries
Dinner	1 chicken breast with brown rice, broccoli, kale and carrots
Pre-bed snack	1 orange

Carbohydrate (g/kg body weight) 5.3	Protein (g/kg body weight) 2.1	Fat (g/kg body weight) 1

Bronze

Beta-alanine: Supplementing with 5g per day of beta-alanine will increase muscle carnosine content of the muscle, therefore increasing buffer capacity, and improve performance of events lasting one to ten minutes. This may allow greater performance during interval training leading to greater adaptations.

Sodium bicarbonate: Supplementing with 0.2–0.3g of sodium bicarbonate ninety minutes prior to interval training sessions may improve performance in those sessions. Alongside this, improvements in the adaptations that enhance lactate transport out of the muscle may be seen.

Further reading

Baar, K. (2006). Training for endurance and strength: lessons from cell signaling. *Medicine and Science in Sports and Exercise*, 38(11), 1939–44. doi:10.1249/01.mss.0000233799.62153.19

Baar, K. (2014). Using molecular biology to maximize concurrent training. *Sports Medicine* (Auckland, N.Z.), 44 Suppl 2, S117–25. doi:10.1007/s40279-014-0252-0

Edge, J., Bishop, D. & Goodman, C. (2006). Effects of chronic NaHCO3 ingestion during interval training on changes to muscle buffer capacity, metabolism, and short-term endurance performance. *Journal of Applied Physiology* (Bethesda, Md. : 1985), 101(3), 918–25. doi:10.1152/japplphysiol.01534.2005

Kendall, K. L., Smith, A. E., Graef, J. L., Fukuda, D. H., Moon, J. R., Beck, T. W., Stout, J. R. (2009). Effects of four weeks of high-intensity interval training and creatine supplementation on critical power and anaerobic working capacity in college-aged men. *Journal of Strength and Conditioning Research / National Strength & Conditioning Association*, 23(6), 1663–9. doi:10.1519/JSC.0b013e3181b1fd1f

Smith, A. E., Walter, A. A., Kendall, K. L., Graef, J. L., Lockwood, C. M., Moon, J. R., Stout, J. R. (2008). Beta-alanine supplementation and high-intensity interval training augments metabolic adaptations and endurance performance in college-aged men. *Journal of the International Society of Sports Nutrition*, 5(Suppl 1), P5. doi:10.1186/1550-2783-5-S1-P5

CHAPTER 5

MAXIMIZING THE ADAPTATIONS TO ENDURANCE TRAINING

At the most basic level the aim of training in endurance sport is to increase the power athletes can produce or the speed they go at for the duration of the event. That performance velocity or power can be thought of as the sum of the aerobic and anaerobic components multiplied by gross mechanical efficiency. Each of these can be broken down into further components.

The aerobic contribution of performance is determined by oxygen uptake at lactate threshold and maximal oxygen uptake. These are further determined by stroke volume, maximum heart rate, haemoglobin content of the blood, aerobic enzyme capacity, and muscle capillary density.

The anaerobic portion of performance is determined by total buffering capacity. Gross mechanical efficiency is determined by the percentage of slow twitch fibres, and anthropometry and elasticity of tendons. Combining all of these is pacing strategy.

Any given exercise session is likely to stimulate adaptations in any one of these factors to ultimately lead to an improvement in sustainable power for a given performance time. In more recent times it has become clear that what you eat also influences the adaptations to exercise. To understand this more, we need to delve deep into the muscle and understand the molecular adaptations to endurance exercise.

As we delve deep into the muscle let me introduce to you the main character of the story. This character is the lynchpin in improving the number of capillaries within your muscles, to increasing the engine of your muscles, the mitochondria and the enzymes that power it. It powers the shift to type I muscle fibres as a consequence of endurance exercise. It is the peroxisome proliferator-activated receptor gamma coactivator 1 alpha, or for simplicity let's use its shortened name, PGC-1 α.

It is ultimately a simplification to suggest that PGC-1 α is the only way the body adapts to endurance exercise, but it does appear to play an essential role and is influenced by nutritional state. If a muscle is artificially stimulated in some way to increase the expression of PGC-1 α, a rise in mitochondria and the corresponding aerobic enzymes is seen. This would lead to a shift towards a greater use of fat as a fuel and a sparing of muscle glycogen. There would be an increase in capillaries, which allow blood to flow through the muscle, providing oxygen, vital nutrients and the removal of waste products. Over time there would be a shift in the muscle fibre type towards a greater proportion of type I fibres,

MAXIMIZING THE ADAPTATIONS TO ENDURANCE TRAINING

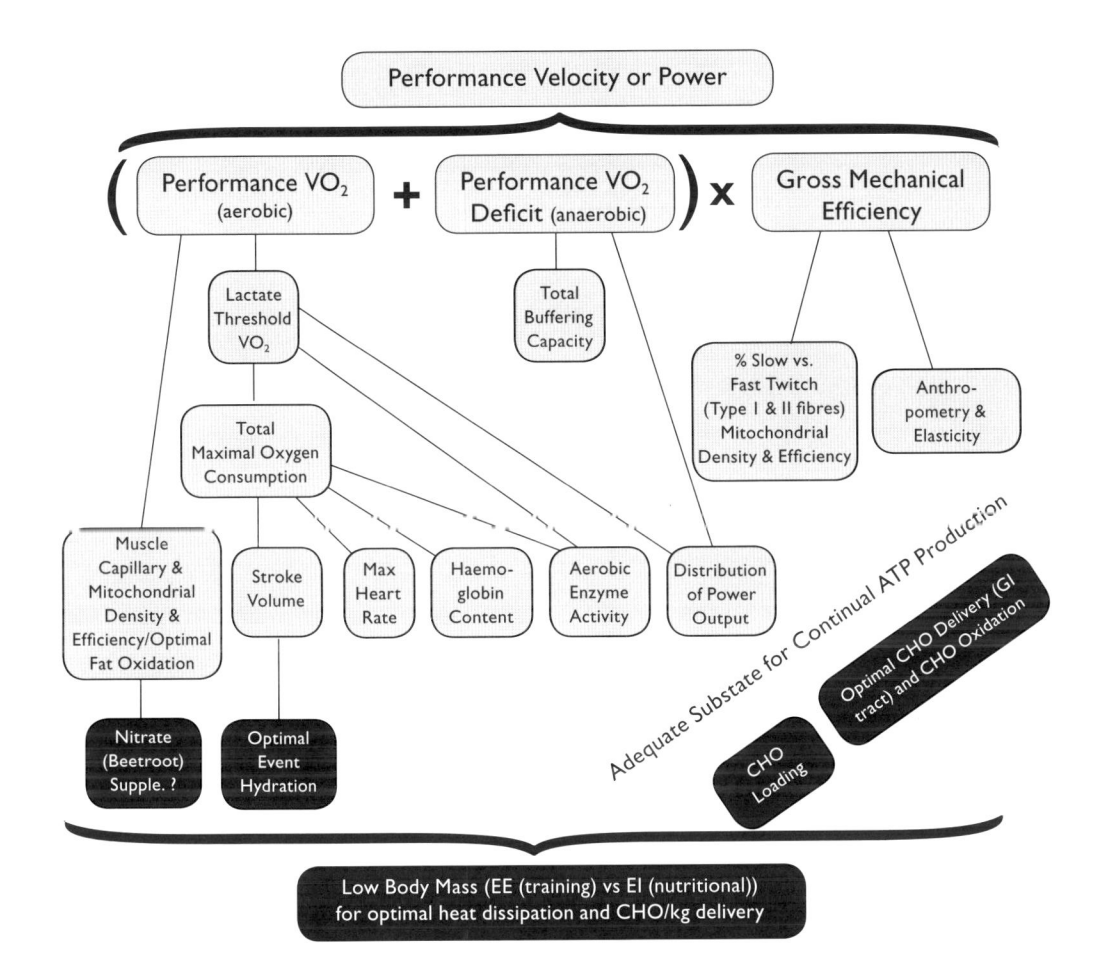

Schematic of how nutrition influences the components of endurance performance (reprinted with permission from Stellingwerf and Spreit, 2014).

which are slow to fatigue and are essential for an endurance athlete.

There are a number of ways in which PGC-1 α can be elevated through different training modes and through dietary interventions. Let's take the most popular training mode for endurance athletes – the long, slow training session – whether it's a cycle, a run or whatever the sport may be. It is the staple training session for any endurance athlete.

When you train long and slow, the repeated muscle contraction leads to an increase in intracellular calcium. Through a cascade of molecular processes this increase in intracellular calcium leads to activation of PGC-1 α, thus leading to favourable adaptations to endurance training.

MAXIMIZING THE ADAPTATIONS TO ENDURANCE TRAINING

Long, slow training will also lead to turnover of energy stores, in particular muscle glycogen. Muscle glycogen is the fuel needed to perform at the desired power for endurance exercise in most cases. However, it seems it is much more than that. It is also a regulator of PGC-1 α through two primary enzymatic pathways, AMPK and p38MAPK. In situations of low muscle glycogen concentrations, both AMPK and p38MAPK are upregulated and stimulate the activation of PGC-1 α. In situations of high muscle glycogen concentrations, the reverse happens.

Muscle glycogen may even bypass PGC-1 α completely. Recent evidence suggests that a reduction in muscle glycogen will stimulate the protein p53. Ok, it's a bit like alphabet soup, and is even more complicated than it sounds. The upshot is that low muscle glycogen concentration leads to favourable endurance adaptations.

Fasted training

Let's get back to the long, slow training session we started with. We see that calcium release during exercise stimulates adaptation to training. As the long, slow training session continues, muscle glycogen will steadily decrease and in some cases become depleted. To match this reduction, fat metabolism will increase so that the muscle can still contract. These two effects will in themselves lead to a positive adaptation to training.

What you eat before long, slow training sessions will have an effect on the muscle glycogen concentration at the beginning of exercise and the rate at which muscle glycogen is used. Ultimately, the meal you eat at this point will affect the adaptive response to exercise. For as long as man has been attempting feats of endurance, the long, slow exercise before breakfast has been a staple of training. Only recently has science caught up with this practice.

It is now clear that training in a fasted state leads to an increase in the ability to use fat as a fuel. This is a consequence of an increase in aerobic enzymes in the muscle. Recent research from the laboratory of Professor Peter Hespel in Belgium has shown this effect. Two groups of ten cyclists trained four times per week, each session lasting sixty to ninety minutes, at approximately 70 per cent VO_2 max, for six weeks. One of the groups ate a carbohydrate-rich breakfast and consumed a sports drink during the training. The second group ate nothing before the ride and consumed only water during the ride.

Let's first take a look at the group that ate breakfast prior to the ride. After the six-week period their VO_2 max had increased by approximately 9 per cent, and the workload at which they burned the most fat as a fuel had increased by 6 per cent. Most importantly, their performance in a one-hour time trial improved by 8 per cent. So what happened to the group who trained fasted each day? Well, they also increased their VO_2 max by 9 per cent. However, the workload at which they maximally used fat as a fuel was increased by 21 per cent. This was a significant and considerable difference compared to the fed group.

If we delve further into the results and look at some other changes in the body, the reason for this becomes clear. Firstly, both groups significantly increased the number of capillaries within the muscle, so there was a better capacity to deliver oxygen and nutrients to their muscles. They both increased the ability to transport carbohydrate into the muscle cells, through an increase in the expression of the glucose transporter 4 (GLUT4) on the cell membranes. However, it was only in the group which fasted before training that there were increases in the aerobic enzymes

MAXIMIZING THE ADAPTATIONS TO ENDURANCE TRAINING

citrate synthase and βhydroxyacyl coenzyme A dehydrogenase (β-HAD). These allow the muscle to be more effective at using fat as a fuel. Despite all of these positive changes the improvements in one-hour time trial performance was the same as if carbohydrate was fed prior to the training sessions. It is likely this length of exercise was not long enough to see a performance effect of fasted training.

Glycogen depletion

Fasted training does seem to have some positive effects on aerobic enzyme adaptations to exercise. Not eating carbohydrates prior to exercise could be one way of enhancing these adaptations. Could another be the deliberate lowering of muscle glycogen prior to exercise training? This was something a research group from the legendary Muscle Research Centre in Copenhagen set out to investigate. They used a laboratory-based exercise model, which involved training the legs only, using a leg-kicking model. On day one of the training week both legs were trained for one hour using the kicking exercise. Following this, both legs rested for two hours. One leg (let's call this one the left one for purposes of clarity) then trained for one hour, while the other rested. On day two the right leg exercised for a further hour, while the left leg rested. This two-day model of exercise continued for five to six days per week for ten weeks.

In essence, both legs got fitter, as evidenced by an increase in maximal workload. However,

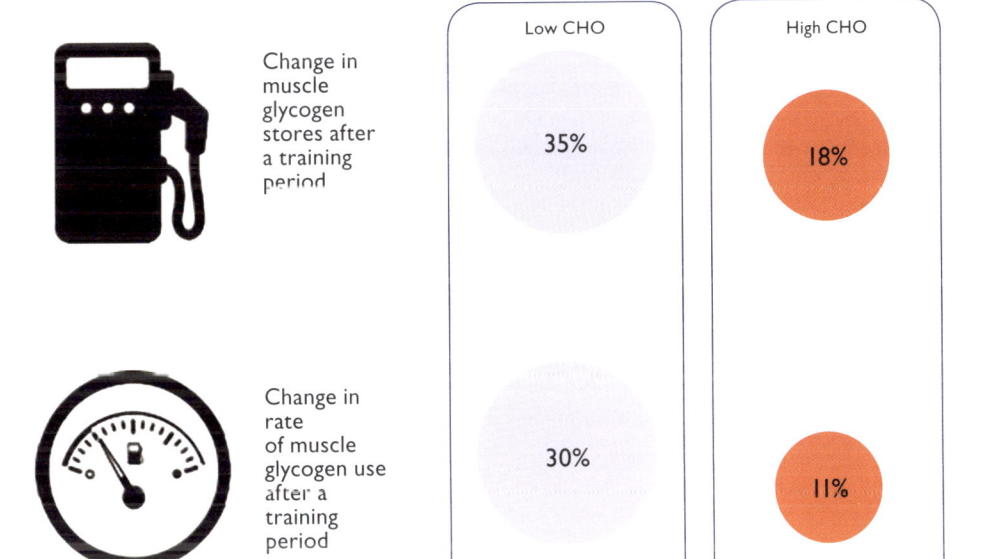

	Low CHO	High CHO
Change in muscle glycogen stores after a training period	35%	18%
Change in rate of muscle glycogen use after a training period	30%	11%

Change in muscle glycogen storage and use after a period of training with high carbohydrate availability or low carbohydrate availability. Muscle glycogen storage is increased, and usage decreased.

when the legs exercised at 90 per cent of this maximal workload until exhaustion, the left leg went for twice as long. One of the major reasons for this was that the left leg had a greater resting muscle glycogen concentration than the right leg. There was also an increase in the aerobic enzymes citrate synthase and β-HAD.

Single leg kicking is a nice model for a laboratory, but bears very little resemblance to real-life activity. This led two research groups, one from the University of Birmingham in the UK and another from Melbourne in Australia, to repeat this using a similar idea but in cyclists. This time each study took two groups of cyclists. One group performed a long, steady-state exercise bout, followed by an interval training session of eight by five minutes of cycling. This took place either one hour after the steady-state exercise or the following morning.

In both studies significant changes in the body's ability to use fat as a fuel were seen when training took place in a glycogen-depleted state. Resting muscle glycogen was increased significantly more in the low-glycogen group, as were the aerobic enzymes citrate synthase and β-HAD. One area of concern was that in both cases the power outputs held in the interval training sessions were significantly lower in the low-glycogen group. This may in the long term be a challenge to training, as essentially training intensity is inhibited by training in a low-glycogen state.

Sleep with low glycogen

A third model of manipulating nutrition to enhance aerobic adaptations to training can be seen in the sleep low-glycogen model. Here, a first exercise bout is completed in the evening. Following this, glycogen is deliberately not replaced, primarily by carbohydrate restriction. The next morning a further exercise bout takes place, prior to any food intake. Subsequently there is a large upregulation of the molecular pathways that stimulate the formation of new aerobic enzymes.

Mitigating against the negative consequences of fasted and depleted training

Whether training in a fasted state, deliberately decreasing muscle glycogen prior to exercise or sleeping in a state of low muscle glycogen, there is a risk involved. Any of these add an extra stress to the body and performing these types of dietary manipulations will lead to a higher risk of injury and illness. Some of the potential negative side effects are:

- An increased strain on the immune system.
- An increase in breakdown of bone, with the potential to lead to a stress fracture with long-term use.
- A loss of muscle mass due to an increase in catabolism.
- A detraining effect due to the reduction in training intensity with low-glycogen training.

One potential way to begin to mitigate against these negative consequences is to consume protein in and around these training sessions. Certainly, prior to fasted training sessions there is evidence that consuming protein will reduce the increase in catabolism seen. It also seems that consuming protein prior to a fasted or low-glycogen training session will not affect the adaptation to that training session.

There are two primary ways to protect against a reduction in training intensity with low-glycogen training. The first is the swilling of carbohydrate around the mouth during the intense training sessions. Simply doing this during the rest periods of an interval training session in a glycogen-depleted state can lead to increases in performance. Likewise, the use of a caffeine dose of approximately 3mg per kg of body weight an hour before the interval session begins will increase power output during the periods of glycogen depletion, although the power output won't quite return to the levels that can be produced in a glycogen-loaded state.

High-fat diets

One of the mechanisms by which low-glycogen training may enhance the adaptation to training is by an increased through-put of fats through the mitochondria. If this is the case, what would be the effect of eating a high-fat diet instead of the usual high-carbohydrate diet of an endurance athlete? This was an approach considered in the late 1990s and early 2000s. During this series of studies it became clear that consuming a high-fat diet for only three days leads to significant changes in metabolism, including:

- A reduction in the use of muscle glycogen as a fuel.
- An increase in the use of fat as a fuel.

The early studies using this model of a high-fat diet were promising. Using models where participants exercised until exhaustion, consuming a high-fat diet led to changes in performance. However, when models using a time trial were analysed, there was no effect compared to a high-carbohydrate diet.

This led to a further model, where for five days a high-fat diet was consumed, followed by one day of a high-carbohydrate diet. Once again, time to exhaustion trials were positive, but no effect was found on time trials. In addition to this, models were performed where high-intensity sprints were included during endurance exercise. This was in an attempt to simulate what is seen in many endurance events, where periods of high-intensity exercise are interspersed within a lower intensity. Using this model, the high-fat diet actually decreased the ability to perform high-intensity exercise. The mechanism for this was through the enzyme pyruvate dehydrogenase (PDH), which is responsible for the conversion of pyruvate to acetyl coA, and thus entry into the Kreb's cycle for oxidation (see Chapter 8 for more on the Kreb's cycle). The downregulation of PDH leads to a reduction in muscle glycogen use, which during high intensity exercise means the metabolic pathways produce ATP at sufficient speed to maintain performance.

It is clear that undertaking training in a glycogen depleted state leads to an increase in the ability to use fat as a fuel and spare muscle glycogen. However, this may come at the expense of training intensity and adaptations to carbohydrate metabolism. The solution may be a mixture of the two models. During a training programme it will be a case of when the training session is long and slow, there should be emphasis on limited carbohydrate intake to maximize endurance adaptations. However, when the training session is about intensity, carbohydrate intake should be the focus. In essence the nutrition intake becomes periodized to the training.

Antioxidants

To mitigate the negative effects of high volumes of endurance training, it is not unusual for high doses of antioxidants to be recommended, particularly vitamins such as C and E. These are normally recommended to support the immune system. However, there may well be consequences to these recommendations in terms of endurance adaptations. Reactive

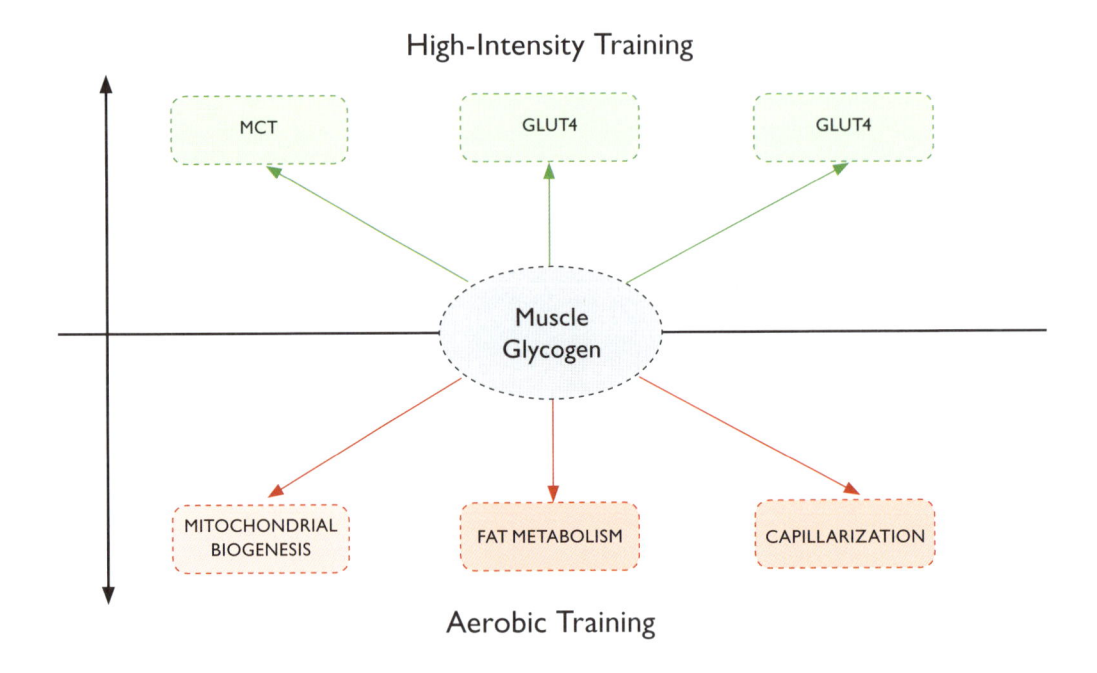

MAXIMIZING THE ADAPTATIONS TO ENDURANCE TRAINING

High-Intensity Training

- MCT
- GLUT4
- GLUT4

Muscle Glycogen

- MITOCHONDRIAL BIOGENESIS
- FAT METABOLISM
- CAPILLARIZATION

Aerobic Training

Role of muscle glycogen in training adaptation. MCT = monocarboxylic transporters, responsible for lactate transport in and out of the muscle amongst other roles; GLUT4 = glucose transporter 4, responsible for the transport of glucose into the muscle; PDH = pyruvate dehydrogenase, a key enzyme linking glycolysis and the Kreb's cycle.

oxygen species (ROS) are produced in the mitochondria during exercise. These ROS are normally quenched by antioxidant enzymes and nutrients, which are naturally produced by the body. They are generally seen as a negative by-product of exercise. However, it appears that a certain amount of ROS are needed to stimulate PGC-1 α.

In a number of studies high doses of synthetic antioxidants including vitamins C and E have been given to athletes undertaking endurance training. The consequence of this supplementation has been a blunting of the increase in mitochondria seen with training. It is likely that there is a dose response to this, with some ROS being needed to promote the adaptation to exercise, but too many can lead to an inhibition of the adaptation to training. Where possible, antioxidants should be obtained from food sources rather than from synthetic supplements. This will reduce the risk of an inhibition of training adaptation.

Protein post-exercise

It is common with resistance exercise to consume protein post-exercise to maximize the adaptation to exercise. While there is less research following endurance exercise, it does appear that ingesting protein post-exercise does lead to an increase in muscle protein synthesis after exercise. Protein synthesis is the marker of formation of new

MAXIMIZING THE ADAPTATIONS TO ENDURANCE TRAINING

proteins in the muscle, either structural or myofibrillar protein, or mitochondrial protein. When protein synthesis response is broken down into these two components, there does seem to be a differing response to protein ingestion after endurance exercise. Consuming protein post-exercise has a clear effect on increasing the structural component of protein synthesis, essentially the building of new muscle fibres. However, the effect of post-exercise protein on the building of new mitochondria seems to be very small, if any.

There does, however, seem to be another positive effect of post-exercise protein intake on the adaptation to endurance exercise. One of the important adaptations to endurance training is an increase in stroke volume to subsequently increase maximal oxygen uptake. One potential mechanism of this increase in stroke volume, through an increase in plasma volume, is an increase in albumin content of the blood to draw fluid into the blood osmotically. This effect can occur relatively quickly. After only five days of aerobic training the cardiovascular changes can be seen. If no protein is consumed post-exercise, plasma volume increases by approximately 4 per cent. However, if protein is consumed

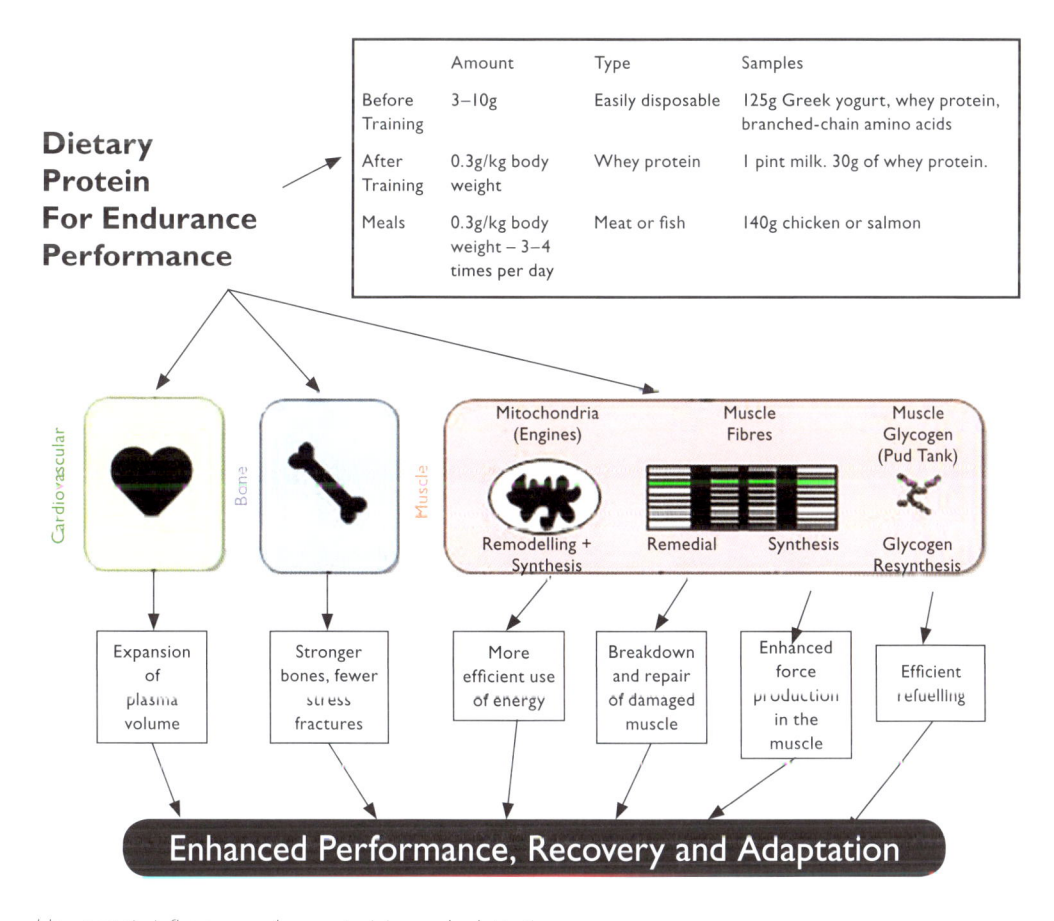

Dietary Protein For Endurance Performance

	Amount	Type	Samples
Before Training	3–10g	Easily disposable	125g Greek yogurt, whey protein, branched-chain amino acids
After Training	0.3g/kg body weight	Whey protein	1 pint milk. 30g of whey protein.
Meals	0.3g/kg body weight – 3–4 times per day	Meat or fish	140g chicken or salmon

How protein influences endurance training and adaptation.

MAXIMIZING THE ADAPTATIONS TO ENDURANCE TRAINING

post-exercise, there is a 7 per cent increase in plasma volume. This seems to follow similar changes in albumin content of the plasma. The functional consequence of this is a lower, slower increase in core temperature at the onset of exercise, and a lower heart rate.

So, how much protein and which type? In terms of aerobic exercise that remains to be determined. However, making inferences from resistance exercise studies, the optimal dose would be 0.3g/kg of body weight post-exercise. The optimal protein type would appear to be whey protein, due to the faster absorption of the amino acid leucine, which is the trigger for many adaptations within the muscle.

Iron

Potentially the most important micronutrient for endurance athletes is the metal iron. Iron status in endurance athletes can be affected by a variety of factors, including dietary intake, training load, gastrointestinal bleeding or haemolysis, which is the process by which red blood cells are broken down and is often found in runners due to the striking of the foot on the ground in a repetitive manner.

How significant the effect of changes in iron status are on endurance performance depends on how severe the iron deficiency is. In individuals who present with iron deficiency anaemia (IDA) there can be a reduction in erythropoiesis, which is the process by which the body produces new red blood cells. As a consequence of this, the concentration of haemoglobin begins to fall in the circulation, and the oxygen-carrying capacity of the blood decreases and negatively affects performance.

A slightly less severe status is when iron deficiency occurs but without anaemia (IDNA). While this process does not affect the oxygen-carrying capacity of the blood, there does seem to be a reduction in enzymatic activity in relation to energy production, ultimately leading to a decrease in performance. Alongside this, IDNA reduces the adaptations seen in response to endurance training.

So if iron deficiency has negative effects on many parts of endurance performance, there is potential for improvements to be made if

> **RESEARCH FOCUS**
>
> **Iron deficiency anaemia and endurance adaptations**
>
> Brownlie et al. (2004) set out to investigate the effects of iron deficiency without anaemia (IDNA) on how female athletes adapt to a four-week block of endurance training. Forty-one untrained female athletes, all of whom presented with IDNA, were randomly assigned to either consume 100mg of ferrous sulphate daily or a placebo.
>
> The total amount of work done in the training load was the same for the two groups. Those who consumed the iron supplement showed a significant improvement in iron status as seen by increases in serum ferritin, whereas in the non-treatment group there was no difference.
>
> The performance tests showed an interesting outcome. While it did not reach significance, there seemed to be a smaller increase in 15km cycling time-trial performance when no treatment was given. Subsequent analysis of the data showed that in all subjects, when serum transferrin receptor was elevated (a marker of iron deficiency), there was no improvement in performance if placebo was given. In those who received treatment a significant improvement in performance was seen.

it can be corrected. A recent meta-analysis published by researchers from St Mary's University in London seems to suggest so. The meta-analysis suggested that iron treatments, either oral or intravenous, led to large improvements in serum transferrin, and had moderate effects on increasing haemoglobin concentration and moderate improvements in VO_2 max.

While it did not seem to matter whether the iron treatment was given orally or through injection, this may be due to smaller numbers of studies investigating intravenous injection of iron in athletes. Studies seem to be suggesting that intravenous injections can be effective in improving iron status.

Iron absorption in the intestine is a complicated process, and absorption is generally poor. Iron comes in two forms, heme and non-heme. Heme iron sources come from animals and non-heme from vegetables or artificial sources. Heme iron is absorbed far more effectively than non-heme.

There are a number of factors that both promote and inhibit iron absorption in the gut. Vitamin C enhances the absorption of iron, while tannins from tea and coffee reduce it.

However, exercise itself can have significant effects on iron absorption, which is tightly regulated and is controlled by a hormone produced in the liver called hepcidin. An increase in hepcidin concentration in the circulation leads to an inhibition of the absorption of iron.

Hepcidin increases in response to inflammation and to exercise itself. The increase in hepcidin post-exercise is driven by increases in the cytokine interleukin-6 (IL-6) and increase in serum iron post-exercise. The increase in serum iron is most likely due to haemolysis, which is particularly relevant for runners where constant foot strike increases the likelihood of this condition.

After running a marathon serum hepcidin concentration can be elevated by up to 27-fold for seventy-two hours after the event. In more regular training just sixty minutes of running leads to an increase in serum hepcidin concentration by up to twenty hours, with peak concentrations apparent after approximately three hours of exercise.

The transient increase in hepcidin post-exercise has consequences for the timing of iron intake, and athletes should avoid the point three hours after a run where hepcidin is elevated. It is suggested that iron supplements be taken either before training or more than four to five hours after training to maximize absorption.

Using the environment to gain endurance adaptations: nutritional considerations

A common approach for endurance athletes is to train in different environmental conditions to evoke a further stress on the body. Commonly this would mean training in either a hot environment or at altitude. Firstly, we will look at how a hot environment can be used to confer benefits for endurance athletes and how nutrition influences the adaptive response.

Heat

For many years it has been the practice that if athletes need to compete in the heat, they train in hot conditions prior to this so that the body can adapt effectively and performance can be maximized. Training in hot conditions covers a whole raft of adaptations that support performance in the heat. Over the first week of so plasma expands to a greater volume, and there is a reduction in sweat sodium concentration and an overall retention of fluid. Subsequent to this, stroke volume increases and heart rate decreases to maintain cardiac output at a given work rate. Over the following week of adaptation, sweating occurs earlier in exercise and at a higher rate, therefore increasing the ability of the body to expel heat. Metabolic efficiency increases and muscle glycogen is spared. Overall, these adaptations lead to a greater ability of the body to maintain core temperature.

Many of the adaptations seen with heat exposure would be of benefit too in temperate conditions, with the adaptations seemingly lasting for one or two weeks after only five days of heat exposure. The overall adaptations to heat acclimatization help to provide the body with a better ability to defend against rises in core temperature. An increase in core temperature is still a component of fatigue even in temperate conditions, mainly due to heat produced through metabolism.

So if heat adaptation can lead to an increase in performance in temperate conditions, how can what an athlete eats or drinks during the period of heat acclimatization help? A study published in 2014 by researchers at the University of Otago may provide an insight. Nine participants undertook a five-day heat acclimation period twice, each time separated by a five-week washout period. During this period of heat acclimatization the participants cycled for ninety minutes for each of the five days in 40°C heat and 60 per cent humidity. During one of the weeks of acclimatization the participants were allowed sufficient fluid during the ninety-minute cycles to maintain hydration status. During the second week the participants were not provided with fluid, therefore inducing a dehydrated state.

Aldosterone is a hormone secreted from the adrenal gland, whose ultimate role is to regulate blood pressure. However, it does this by regulating water and electrolyte balance. An increase in aldosterone ultimately leads to a greater retention of fluid. When the participants performed the period of acclimatization in a dehydrated state, aldosterone increased by a greater extent across the exercise bout than when exercise was performed in a hydrated state.

As a consequence of this greater increase in aldosterone, there was a greater expansion of plasma volume in response to exercise. There appeared to be a greater forearm blood flow, indicating a greater ability to dissipate heat with acclimatization in a dehydrated state and a trend towards a lower core temperature at the end of an exercise heat-stress test with dehydrated acclimatization. Overall these data give an indication that restricting fluid during heat acclimatization will lead to greater adaptations to the acclimatization and ultimately lead to greater performance improvements.

Altitude

So heat exposure and deliberate dehydrating can lead to positive adaptations to enhance endurance performance. How can nutrition and altitude exposure lead to adaptations that will enhance endurance performance? Altitude training leads to a range of positive adaptations, which can result in improvements in endurance performance at sea level. These include an increase in red cell mass and therefore a better ability to transport oxygen within the circulation, an improved ability to cope with changes in pH within the muscle, and increases in oxidative enzymes.

Throughout a period of altitude training a number of interventions can be put in place to enhance the adaptive response. Firstly, more than four weeks prior to the altitude training, serum ferritin should be assessed as a marker of iron status. Research has shown that if serum ferritin is low, and therefore a marker of a deficiency in iron status, adaptations to the altitude exposure will not occur.

If serum ferritin is low, interventions should be put in place to correct the deficiency, as outlined earlier in this chapter.

Upon altitude exposure the first nutritional consideration should be to prevent the athlete from getting ill. Altitude itself provides a challenge to the intestine in particular. As we saw in Chapter 1, the intestine is the first barrier to infection. Exercise itself provides a challenge to intestinal permeability and integrity, and can lead to an increase in the tight junction space between the intestinal cells. Essentially, the intestine becomes more porous. Added to this the altitude exposure also causes an increase in intestinal permeability. This is due to reduced oxygen availability, and therefore causes a stress on the intestine.

There are a number of interventions that can help at this point to reduce intestinal permeability. Although none have been tested specifically in altitude exposure, probiotics, colostrum and glutamine supplementation have been shown to reduce intestinal permeability. Colostrum and glutamine supplementation have both been shown to reduce the increase in intestinal permeability due to exercise.

Once it is ensured that an athlete is well, the next challenge an athlete faces is a reduction in muscle mass due to altitude exposure. Much of the research is aimed at an altitude higher than usually seen for altitude training, which is normally between 1,200m and 2,500m. When exposed to altitude there is an increased turnover of amino acids within the muscle, with increases in muscle breakdown and synthesis seen. However, synthesis is limited by amino acid availability, and this must come from either further tissue breakdown or from diet. Therefore, ensuring adequate dietary protein intake is important with altitude exposure to allow athletes to maintain muscle mass.

Athletes should aim to consume four to six meals containing 0.3g of protein per kg of body weight. This will provide substrate for the increased turnover of amino acids and protect muscle mass. Athletes should have a plan to meet these needs, as appetite is suppressed at altitude and they may not freely choose to consume adequate food.

RESEARCH FOCUS

Hypoxic exposure and protein synthesis

The legendary research group of Bengt Saltin from the University of Copenhagen undertook research looking at exposing nine male participants who lived at sea level to an altitude of 4,559m for seven to nine days. Stable isotope tracers were used to assess both muscle protein synthesis and breakdown at sea level and at altitude.

The rate of protein synthesis was increased by approximately 9 per cent compared to sea level, with protein breakdown increasing by a similar amount. The increases in both synthesis and breakdown came from the structural or myofibrillar component of muscle, suggesting a reason why muscle mass loss may occur at altitude.

A major adaptation to altitude exposure is an increase in erythropoiesis – to ultimately increase red cell mass and the oxygen-carrying capacity of the blood. At a molecular level one of the key triggers for erythropoiesis is an increase in the expression of hypoxia inducible factor-1 α (HIF-1 α). An increase in HIF-1α leads to a cascade of molecular signals that ultimately result in erythropoiesis. There is also an increase in absorption of iron in the intestine, as HIF-1α expression leads to a decrease in circulating hepcidin concentrations. Hepcidin is the hormone that

MAXIMIZING THE ADAPTATIONS TO ENDURANCE TRAINING

Table 5.1 Iron-containing foods.

Food	Handy Measures	Weight (g)	Iron Content (mg)
Meat, Fish & Alternatives			
Baked beans in tomato sauce	1 small tin	225	3.2
Beef mince, stewed	Small portion	150	4.7
Bolognese sauce	Average portion	200	4.8
Chilli con carne	Average portion	200	4.4
Lean roast lamb	Small portion	100	1.7
Liver	Small portion	50	6.4
Liver pâté low fat	Average on slice of bread	50	3.1
Moussaka	Average portion	300	3.3
Pilchards in tomato sauce	Half small can	100	2.7
Red salmon, canned	Large portion	100	1.4
Sardines in tomato sauce	Large portion in sandwich	50	2.3
Shepherd's pie	Average portion	300	3.6
Fruit & Vegetables			
Apricots (ready soaked)	10 (snack pack size)	50	3.4
Figs, dried	4 figs	75	3.2
Spinach, boiled	Average serving	100	1.7
Bread, other Cereals & Potatoes			
All-Bran/Bran Buds	Medium portion	50	6.0
Bread, wholemeal	3 medium sliced	100	2.6
Jacket potato	Large	200	1.4
Muesli, not crunchy	Small portion	50	2.8
Shredded Wheat	2 pieces	50	2.0
Weetabix	2 biscuits	50	3.8
Weetaflakes	Small portion	25	2.9
Wholemeal pitta bread	1 small	75	2.0
Wholemeal roll	1 roll	50	1.7
Miscellaneous			
Rich fruit cake	Average portion	75	1.4
Tahini (sesame seed paste)	1 heaped teaspoon	25	2.6
Toasted teacake/currant bun	1 teacake/1 bun	50	1.2
Plain Digestive biscuit	3 biscuits	50	1.6

regulates the absorption of iron in the intestine.

One of the first considerations is to ensure that there is sufficient nutrient intake to help build the new red blood cells needed for the adaptation. Three nutrients in particular are key to achieving this. Obviously there is a greater need for iron in the diet, as can be seen by the greater rate of absorption. Alongside this, B-vitamins and folic acid should be increased as they are also part of the process of production of new red blood cells.

Hypoxic exposure also affects redox balance within the body. Redox balance is the continual balance of oxidative stress and antioxidant status. Hypoxic exposure leads to an increase in oxidative stress and a general trend to a decrease in antioxidant status during the same period. The increase in oxidative stress appears to play an important role in promoting the adaptations to altitude training. Oxidative stress promotes the expression of HIF-1α.

But why might antioxidant status decrease with altitude exposure? A simple reason could be a poor dietary intake of key antioxidants such as vitamins A, C and E. Researchers from a French research group exposed six elite male cross-country skiers to living at a simulated altitude of 2,500–3,500m, while training at 1,200m. Alongside this, dietary assessments took place to look at food intake.

Altitude exposure increased oxidative stress, but at the same time there was a trend towards a decrease in antioxidant status. Alongside this, biomarker analysis showed decreases in the food-based antioxidants lycopene and β-carotene. Vitamin E, a potent dietary antioxidant, was only 53 per cent of the sedentary Recommended Dietary Allowance (RDA) – clearly a low intake, particularly given athletes' need for a higher one. Vitamin A and C intakes were only just below the RDA, though again intakes for athletes may need to be higher, particularly for vitamin C. The relatively low vitamin A and E intake may be due to the low fat intake in these athletes, as they are fat-soluble vitamins.

The research from the French group clearly shows that dietary intake was inadequate in these athletes and was likely to contribute to the decrease in antioxidant status throughout altitude exposure. Therefore, ensuring adequate micronutrient intake during altitude exposure is crucial.

However, care should be taken in providing mega-doses of antioxidants during altitude exposure, as oxidative stress is important in the adaptation process. Supplementation with high doses of vitamins or other antioxidants may blunt the adaptation to altitude exposure. Taking an approach of increasing dietary intake of micronutrients should be adequate.

Training at altitude can lead to a decrease in performance of high-intensity exercise. One possible solution to the reduction in exercise intensity could be to supplement with dietary nitrates to enhance performance. Research from the research group of Professor Andy Jones at the University of Exeter shows an improvement in performance in hypoxic conditions when supplemented with 9.3 mmol of nitrates, in the form of 0.75l of beetroot juice over the twenty four hours prior to exercise in hypoxia. Decreases in performance due to hypoxic exposure were attenuated, and participants were able to perform as well in hypoxia as at sea level. This might provide a technique by which intensity can be maintained while training at altitude.

Summary

- Performance velocity or power in endurance sports is the sum of the aerobic and anaerobic components of energy production multiplied by gross mechanical efficiency.
- Aerobic contribution to performance is determined by oxygen uptake at lactate threshold and maximal oxygen uptake.
- The anaerobic component is determined by total buffering capacity.
- Gross mechanical efficiency is determined by the percentage of slow twitch fibres, anthropometry and the elasticity of tendons.
- PGC-1α is a molecular trigger for many training adaptations related to endurance performance within the muscle. It plays a role in determining the number of

capillaries in the muscle, increases mitochondrial density and aerobic enzyme production, and leads to fibre type determination. It is not the only process to do this, but is influenced by training and diet.
- PGC-1α is increased by a variety of different ways depending on the training session.

Gold
Fasted training: Performing long, slow training sessions in the fasted state will lead to greater adaptations in fat metabolism than if performed in the fed state. This is a method that has been used for many decades by endurance athletes. Consuming protein prior to this session will not inhibit the adaptations to the training session.

Iron: Adequate iron status is essential for adaptation to endurance training. Iron supplementation is only really needed if a deficiency is identified. Meat-based sources of iron provide better absorption than vegetable sources for the general diet. Low iron status may also be a sign of poor recovery practices.

Silver
Glycogen depletion: Performing a training session prior to a high-intensity exercise session, with minimal food in between, will improve some adaptations to endurance training.

Sleep with low glycogen: A further model to enhance adaptations to endurance training is to perform a training session in the evening, restrict carbohydrates post-exercise, and then perform a further training session the following morning.

Protein post-exercise: Consuming 0.3g of protein per kg of body weight post-exercise will maximize any increases in protein synthesis needed. It will also help promote adaptations in plasma volume and therefore cardiovascular function, which may be needed.

Dehydration: Deliberately restricting fluid intake while in a period of heat adaptation may enhance the cardiovascular adaptations to heat exposure.

Bronze
Mouth-swilling and caffeine during fasted/depleted training: Swilling carbohydrate around the mouth or consuming 1–3mg of caffeine per kg of body weight thirty to sixty minutes prior to a training session may help to maintain intensity and reduce perception of effort during the training session.

High-fat diet: There seems to be some evidence that a high-fat diet improves many of the aerobic adaptations to endurance training. However, doing this will reduce the ability to produce high levels of force. Glycolysis will also be inhibited.

Nutrition for altitude training: Athletes should be aware of the greater protein needs at altitude, along with being mindful of consuming foods high in iron, folic acid and B vitamins to promote red blood cell formation.

Further reading

Goto, M., Okazaki, K., Kamijo, Y., Ikegawa, S., Masuki, S., Miyagawa, K. & Nose, H. (2010). Protein and carbohydrate supplementation during 5-day aerobic training enhanced plasma volume expansion and thermoregulatory adaptation in young men. *Journal of Applied Physiology* (Bethesda, Md.: 1985), 109(4), 1247–55. doi:10.1152/japplphysiol.00577.2010

Table 5.2 Example diet plan for Chapter 5.

Meal	Food
Breakfast	3-egg omelette with mushrooms, peppers and cheese 125g pot of Greek yogurt 1 cup of coffee with 2 espresso shots
During exercise – 3–4 hours of exercise	Water
Post-exercise	20g of whey protein with 35g of carbohydrates, made with 400ml of milk
Lunch	1 tin of tuna with a baked sweet potato and a mixed salad
Snack	2 slices of wholemeal bread with almond butter and a handful of berries
Dinner	1 chicken breast with brown rice, broccoli, kale and carrots
Pre-bed snack	125g tub of Greek yogurt

Carbohydrate (g/kg body weight)	Protein (g/kg body weight)	Fat (g/kg body weight)
3.6	2.3	1.3

Hawley, J. A. & Morton, J. P. (2014). Ramping up the signal: promoting endurance training adaptation in skeletal muscle by nutritional manipulation. *Clinical and Experimental Pharmacology & Physiology*, 41(8), 608–13. doi:10.1111/1440-1681.12246

Holm, L., Haslund, M. L., Robach, P., van Hall, G., Calbet, J. A. L., Saltin, B. & Lundby, C. (2010). Skeletal muscle myofibrillar and sarcoplasmic protein synthesis rates are affected differently by altitude-induced hypoxia in native lowlanders. *PloS One*, 5(12), e15606. doi:10.1371/journal.pone.0015606

Moore, D. R., Camera, D. M., Areta, J. L. & Hawley, J. A. (2014). Beyond muscle hypertrophy: why dietary protein is important for endurance athletes. *Applied Physiology, Nutrition, and Metabolism = Physiologie Appliquée, Nutrition et Métabolisme*, 39(9), 987–97. doi:10.1139/apnm-2013-0591

Stellingwerff, T. & Spriet, L. L. (2014). Introduction. Nutritional triggers to adaptation and performance. *Applied Physiology, Nutrition, and Metabolism = Physiologie Appliquée, Nutrition et Métabolisme*, 39(9), v–vi. doi:10.1139/apnm-2014-0217

CHAPTER 6

NUTRITION AND THE BRAIN

How many sports are determined by the ability to make the right decision, at the right time? To react to a stimulus, and to learn and perform a skill? My guess is you can think of many situations like this. So much of sports nutrition has focused on how nutrients influence the muscle, and the cardiovascular system at a push, yet very little has focused on how nutrients interact with the brain to influence skill- or decision-based outcomes.

Maintaining brain function under conditions of fatigue

Much of the research into the effects of different nutrients on sporting performance has focused on cognitive function under physical stress. Normally this has involved performing certain tasks related to brain function at the end of a period of physical exercise and how those nutrients prevent a decrease in brain function.

The most common nutrients that have been investigated with respect to cognitive function are the branched-chain amino acids: leucine, isoleucine and valine. These have been heavily linked to delaying central fatigue through a series of hypotheses postulated by the legendary biochemist Eric Newsholme from the University of Oxford. The hypothesis was based around increases in serotonin, where increases in serotonin within the brain were seen as one of the potential causes of fatigue.

Serotonin is synthesized from the amino acid tryptophan, and when tryptophan concentrations are increased within the blood then more serotonin is produced in the brain, thus causing fatigue. The transport of tryptophan across the blood–brain barrier occurs in competition with the three branched-chain amino acids. However, during prolonged exercise the plasma concentrations of the branched-chain amino acids decrease due to them being oxidized to produce energy. This decrease in circulating branched-chain amino acids leads to an increase in transport of tryptophan across the blood–brain barrier, increased serotonin production and therefore fatigue.

One intervention suggested to prevent this decrease in branched-chain amino acids is supplementation with the branched-chain amino acids themselves. Early studies in rodent models of exercise seemed to be promising. However, human research showing an increase in performance during prolonged exercise with branched-chain amino acid supplementation has not been as positive.

A handful of studies have investigated the effects of branched-chain amino acid supplementation during prolonged exercise and measures of cognitive function throughout the period of exercise. These studies have suggested that during prolonged exercise, such as a 30km run, branched-chain amino acid supplementation will improve an athlete's attention, but does very little for their ability to perform less demanding cognitive tasks such as short-term memory or mathematical tasks. It seems there may be some benefit to supplementing with branched-chain amino acids to improve cognitive function if there is a period of physical stress involved too.

It is clear from current research on how food and individual nutrients influence brain function that one challenge the research faces is how cognitive function is measured. There has been very little attention placed on sport-specific measures of cognitive function, and many measures are laboratory-based with assumptions having to be made to transfer these to sporting performance.

Potentially, there are a number of aspects of cognitive and skill performance that could be influenced by different nutrients. At a skill-based level there could be the potential to influence skill performance, either the smaller fine motor movements or larger gross movements. Alongside this, changes in coordination of these skills and movements may be seen. Improvements in reaction time were visible, too.

The food we eat could influence our ability to maintain our attention focus and be vigilant over a period of time. The food could increase our alertness and allow us to improve our memory both over the short and long term.

As we saw with branched-chain amino acid supplementation, one potential mechanism to influence these areas of cognitive function is to try to alter or maintain the biochemistry of the brain and nervous system. While the idea of supplementing with branched-chain amino acids is a nice one, the practical evidence is not so prevalent. However, one nutrient that can have significant effects on the function of the brain is glucose, the most simple of nutrients and one that has been mentioned many times throughout this book.

Blood glucose

We know that blood glucose provides a major fuel for the muscle to function effectively. It is also well known that the brain relies heavily on blood glucose as a fuel. Brain cells have a high energy demand; in fact they generally need double the energy of a cell in any other part of the body as they are always active, even during periods of rest and sleep. Nerve transmission itself accounts for half of the brain's energy demand, and around 10 per cent of the whole body's energy demands.

During tasks that demand high levels of concentration the brain's use of glucose can be phenomenal. While much of the research conducted in this area has been with rats, specific areas of the brain see large increases in glucose use in response to a task that requires significant concentration. The amount of glucose the brain uses appears to increase with age, too.

The simplest way to demonstrate the effects of glucose on cognitive function is to look at the effect of performing various cognitive tasks before or after breakfast. A study from the University of Toronto gave older adults either a cereal- and fruit-based breakfast or water only prior to a memory-based task. Performance of the cognitive tasks was improved by 25 per cent after breakfast was given.

The ability to supply glucose to the brain during difficult cognitive tasks is important, not only due to the increased demand for glucose during these tasks but due to there being a very limited storage of carbohydrate in the brain. Maintaining a steady blood-glucose concentration is important, too. Large increases in blood glucose, say after ingesting a sugar drink, may give some immediate benefits to brain function, but will have very little effect in the long term as insulin

NUTRITION AND THE BRAIN

secretion after the sugary drink ingestion will lead to a decrease in blood glucose.

Supplementation with carbohydrate seems to be most effective when there is a high cognitive load. Two tests commonly used to measure memory and concentration are serial 7s and serial 3s. These simply involve counting back from 100 in either 7s or 3s. Serial 7s is seen as a test with a high cognitive load and serial 3s less so. Studies have shown that supplementing with carbohydrate during tests of serial 7s improves performance on the test, but does very little on tests of serial 3s.

This is unsurprising as we know that the brain uses glucose at an increasing rate as the difficulty of the task increases. Therefore, it is also unsurprising that when prolonged exercise is performed, which is known to also decrease blood glucose, carbohydrate supplementation also improves cognitive performance after the prolonged exercise tasks.

Apart from being used as a fuel by the brain, carbohydrate may influence cognitive function in two ways. Firstly, by reducing the increase in brain serotonin. As outlined earlier, one hypothesis of central fatigue is an increase in free tryptophan circulating in the blood, crossing the blood–brain barrier and therefore causing the synthesis of serotonin. Normally tryptophan circulates around the bloodstream attached to albumin. However, during prolonged exercise there is an increase in circulating free fatty acids, as they are mobilized from adipose tissue for use as a fuel. This

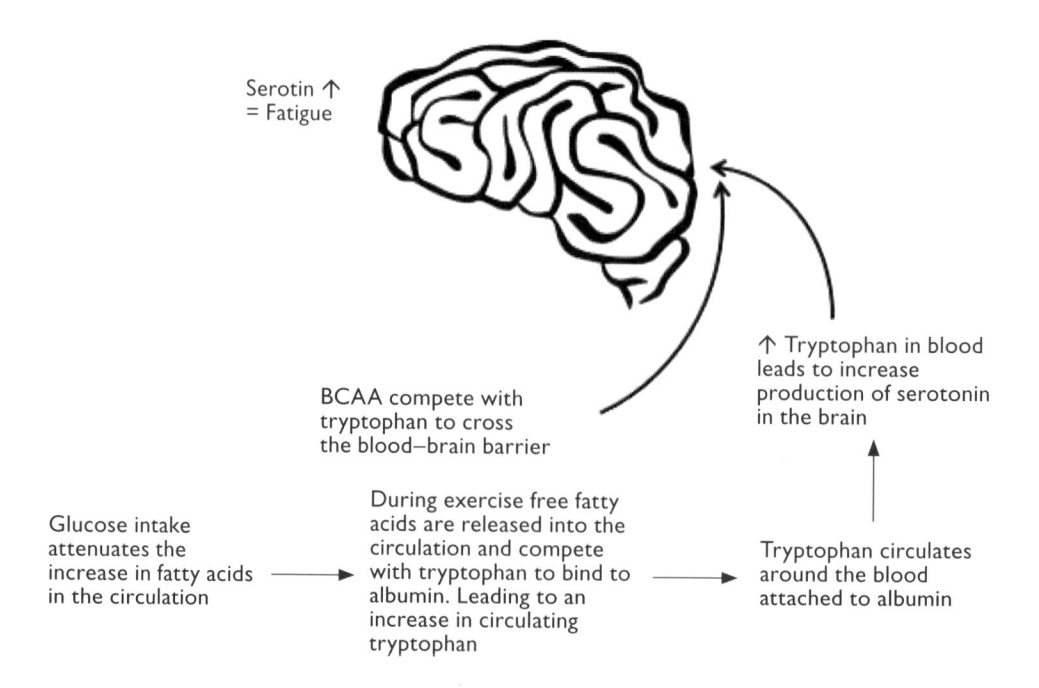

Schematic of how nutrients might influence brain serotonin production.

NUTRITION AND THE BRAIN

increase in circulating free fatty acid concentration leads to direct competition with tryptophan to bind with albumin, leading to an increase in free tryptophan. However, supplementation with carbohydrates during prolonged exercise attenuates the increase in free fatty acids in the blood and therefore more tryptophan remains bound to albumin.

A second role for carbohydrates in brain function could be the importance of carbohydrate availability for synthesis of acetylcholine. Acetylcholine is one of the key neurotransmitters and any decrease in synthesis can inhibit cognitive function.

A further way for carbohydrate to influence brain performance could be through the sensing of carbohydrate in the mouth. It has become clear over the last ten years or so that there are sensors within the mouth that respond to the presence of carbohydrate. This sensing of carbohydrate can lead to an improvement in performance of events lasting up to one hour.

While there is very little evidence that mouth rinsing with carbohydrate improves motor skill performance, brain imaging techniques seem to show activation of areas of the brain associated with motor skill function along with reward. This could be an interesting development in the coming years.

Caffeine

You wake up, the alarm having startled you out of bed. Your first thought is to put the kettle on and have a good cup of tea or strong, freshly ground coffee. For many people, tea and coffee is a key part of their daily food intake. The two have caffeine in common, possibly the most popular drug used worldwide.

Caffeine is associated with improving brain function and performance. It is well known that caffeine can delay fatigue in both short-term high-intensity exercise and endurance exercise. An increasing amount of evidence is supporting the use of caffeine for skill performance, too.

Across a number of different skill-based sports, caffeine has been shown to improve performance. This seems particularly true in team-based sports where an amount of physical fatigue accumulates due to the nature of the sport. Research has shown that doses in the region of 4–6mg of caffeine per kg of body weight taken prior to the start of a match can improve passing accuracy in both football and rugby, along with dribbling ability in field hockey. For many of these research studies, skill performance was improved by caffeine in the second half in particular.

Caffeine intake has also been shown to improve reaction time and attention to both simple and complex laboratory-based tasks. However, it is not always clear whether caffeine ingestion makes you more accurate. Imagine doing a test where you have to respond to a given letter on the screen, but ignore others. You are likely to respond to the stimulus faster when you have taken caffeine before the task, but may not always respond more accurately.

What about more complex tasks of attention? The Rapid Visual Information Processing test is one that is used in laboratories to assess complex task performance. On a screen in front of the participant, single digit numbers flash up on the screen at a rate of 100 per minute, and the participant must detect different patterns in the numbers. On a test such as this, caffeine can improve overall performance, reaction time and accuracy.

Caffeine may not always be positive for performance. For some individuals caffeine can lead to an increase in anxiety and tension, and impair fine motor control. I am sure many

NUTRITION AND THE BRAIN

people who drink coffee, and certainly those who drink a little too much in a day, will have experienced the shakes. As you can imagine, when your hands are shaking too much, performing fine motor tasks like shooting or archery will be difficult.

There seems to be very little evidence to suggest that high doses of caffeine are needed to provide an effect. Very small-dose response studies have been conducted on how caffeine can improve cognitive performance, and it seems that doses as small as 2–3mg per kg of body weight will be effective.

So how does caffeine work to influence the brain? When you consume caffeine, whether in pure form or in coffee or tea, it is quickly absorbed in the gastrointestinal tract, where it enters the bloodstream and can remain for between two and a half and ten hours, depending on the individual. Caffeine's primary mechanism of action is by acting as an antagonist to adenosine receptors in the brain. Adenosine receptors play a role in the sleep/wake cycle, with an increase seen throughout the day and a decrease at night. As caffeine binds to these receptors, adenosine cannot. Therefore, alertness can be maintained for longer.

The effect of caffeine on cognitive function could be enhanced by the addition of the amino acid L-theanine. L-theanine is a naturally occurring amino acid, which can be found in particular in tea, especially green tea. When taken in conjunction with caffeine it seems that L-theanine can improve attention, whereas when taken alone it seems to have little effect.

Polyphenols and flavanols

Would you believe that chocolate can allow your brain to work more effectively? Maybe that chocolate bar at three in the afternoon works after all to get you through the working day. Unfortunately, that's not quite the case, but it seems that the humble cocoa bean, and extracts of it, can lead to improvements in brain function. This is because cocoa beans are naturally high in micronutrients called flavanols, which along with the micronutrients appear to influence brain function.

When extracts of cocoa beans have been supplemented prior to complex cognitive tasks there have been significant improvements in attention during these laboratory-based cognitive tasks. Alongside this, when good-quality dark chocolate was consumed prior to a cognitive task (compared to white chocolate, which contains very few flavanols) there were improvements in visual function and memory across tasks.

A similar story begins to appear across a number of different foods that contain large amounts of micronutrients, such as poly-phenols and flavonoids. Improvements in cognitive function appear across other substances, such as blueberries and sage or herbal preparations such as gingko biloba and Rhodiola rosea. In some cases they have been supplemented over a two-week period, others only acutely. Dosing, therefore, is unclear.

So what is it about these foods, and their extracts, that improve cognitive function? Mechanisms seem unclear, although the most likely explanation is that all of these substances seem to increase blood flow to the brain. Brain imaging studies after ingestion of cocoa flavanols provide an interesting insight into the potential mechanisms by which these substances may influence brain function. When cocoa flavanols were fed for five consecutive days, the brain imaging scans showed a significant increase in blood flow to the brain. This increase in blood flow seems to come through the influence of polyphenols on the nitric oxide vasodilation pathways, which leads to the possibility of high nitrate-containing foods, such as beetroot juice, influencing cognitive function.

Creatine

Creatine is better known for supporting high-intensity exercise performance and hypertrophy than for its effect on the brain. However, throughout the early part of the twenty-first century evidence has been growing to show the effect that creatine supplementation has on cognitive performance. Much of this research started in clinical settings looking at the role of high-energy phosphates, and more specifically phosphocreatine, in diseases such as depression and schizophrenia.

So if you supplement with creatine, is there an increase in phosphocreatine concentrations in the brain? Researchers from Harvard University used magnetic imaging techniques to investigate the effects of creatine monohydrate supplementation for an initial seven-day loading period and a further seven-day maintenance period. Over this period there was a 3.4 per cent increase in phosphocreatine concentration in the brain. So it seems that creatine supplementation can increase the creatine content of the brain.

At present, outside of clinical situations this does not seem to lead to too many performance outcomes. From these clinical situations and from sleep deprivation studies it is clear that the creatine content of the brain does decrease, and supplementation with creatine will restore creatine concentrations in the brain.

Christian Cook and colleagues from a number of British universities investigated the effects of acute creatine supplementation on rugby skill performance under conditions of sleep deprivation. This was compared to the effects of caffeine, with both being provided 90 minutes prior to the start of the skill task. Sleep deprivation decreased performance on the skill task, whereas both caffeine and creatine prevented this drop in performance – a promising development for creatine that might lead to improved skill performance in certain situations.

Tyrosine

The amino acid tyrosine is a precursor for dopamine production, as well as catecholamine production. It is commonly suggested that tyrosine can improve cognitive function, because during situations of stress there is the possibility that the body cannot synthesize sufficient neurotransmitters. As tyrosine is a precursor to these neurotransmitters, there is therefore a potential to influence cognitive performance.

In animal-based studies this does appear to be the case. When in mentally stressful situations, tyrosine will improve cognitive performance. However, human studies are scarce, if not promising. It seems there is potential for supplementation of 100–300mg of tyrosine to influence cognitive performance, although it seems it is only the case in situations of high physical or mental stress. More research needs to be conducted in this area.

Long-term nutrient intake

There appears to be a number of nutrients, therefore, which given over the short term can improve various aspects of cognitive function. However, two food groups over the long term seem to influence brain function. Much of this research has come from how food might influence development of illnesses such as dementia and Alzheimer's.

The first is potentially one of the most

NUTRITION AND THE BRAIN

forgotten food groups: fruit and vegetables. We all know they are important, yet many of us don't consume anywhere near enough of them. It appears they are not only important for our general health, but fruit and vegetable intake over the long term has significant effects on our brain function.

Epidemiological studies have shown that those who contract Alzheimer's are more likely to have had a lower intake of fruit and vegetables on a daily basis than those who don't develop the condition. Consuming fewer than two portions of fruit and vegetables per day leads to a significant decrease in memory and overall brain function. This is in healthy individuals, never mind those who may have some form of disease.

Vegetables in particular seem to be important in decreasing cognitive decline with ageing. Long-term consumption of cruciferous vegetables in particular seems to be linked with better cognitive performance. So eating those brussels sprouts, broccoli and cauliflower could really be important where brain performance is concerned.

What is so potent about fruit and vegetables for them to be so important for our brain? Their vitamin C content may be key. Vitamin C has been shown to accumulate in neurons and act as a scavenger for free radicals. These free radicals can decrease cognitive performance, especially over a long period of time. The accumulation of vitamin C in neurons will also spare alpha tocopherol, or vitamin

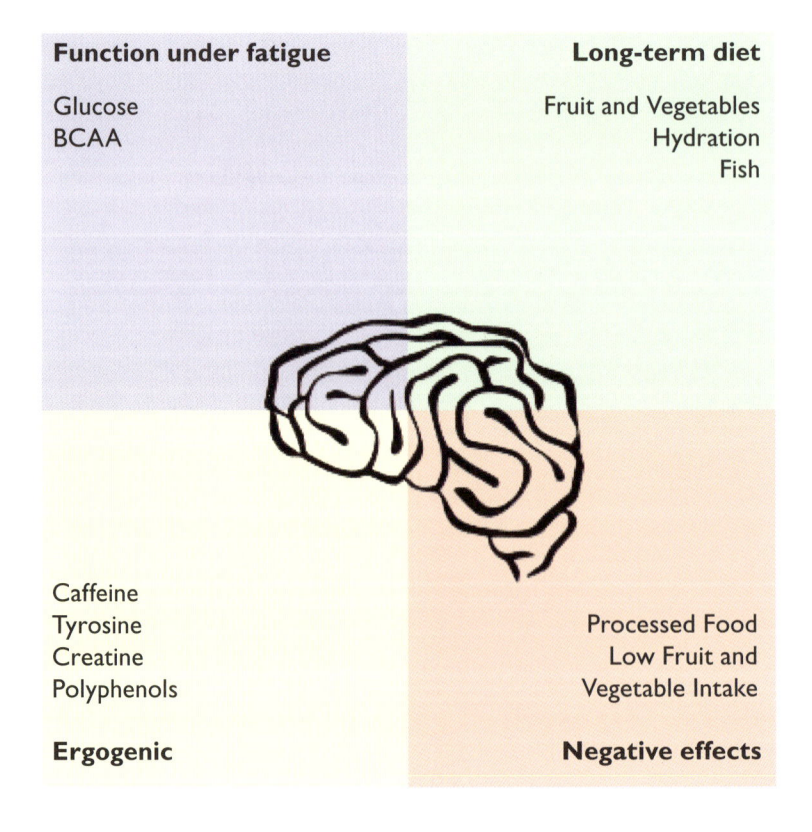

Function under fatigue	**Long-term diet**
Glucose	Fruit and Vegetables
BCAA	Hydration
	Fish
Caffeine	
Tyrosine	Processed Food
Creatine	Low Fruit and
Polyphenols	Vegetable Intake
Ergogenic	**Negative effects**

Nutrient effects on the brain.

NUTRITION AND THE BRAIN

E to many of us. Vitamin E is a fat-soluble vitamin, and as the brain is a fat-rich environment, vitamin E is likely to play a key role in effective brain function. Vitamin C is also important in the synthesis of various neurotransmitters, giving further support to the importance of fruit and vegetables for brain function.

Of course, fruit and vegetables contain many other nutrients that are likely to support effective brain functioning, including B vitamins and of course polyphenols, covered earlier in the chapter.

The second food type to have an effect on cognitive performance is fish, particular oily fish such as salmon and mackerel. Many studies have shown a correlation between fish intake and maintenance of cognitive function in ageing.

Oily fish provide a good source of the omega 3 fatty acids eicosapentaenoic acid (EPA) and docosahexaenoic acid (DHA). While minimal human studies have been conducted, there is some evidence for the role of DHA in maintaining brain function and promoting skill learning. One human study in athletes showed that 2.2g per day of omega 3 supplementation for twenty-one days reduced reaction time to a stimulus, with increases in speed of signal travel from the brain to the muscles.

Summary

- Many sports are determined by making the right decision or by reacting to a stimulus, yet much of sports nutrition has been focused on the muscle. Nutrients can also influence brain function.
- Nutrients can influence brain function by delaying fatigue and therefore allowing the brain to still function under conditions of fatigue.
- Food and the nutrients within them can influence brain function by directly altering the brain biochemistry or by increasing blood flow to the brain.
- However, measuring brain function is incredibly difficult.
- Blood glucose concentration potentially has the largest effect on brain function. A lowering of blood glucose concentration will lead to a decrease in the fuel available for the brain to use.

Gold

Carbohydrate supplementation: During periods of heavy cognitive demand, supplementing with 30–60g of carbohydrate will improve cognitive performance. Having a high-carbohydrate, low-glycaemic index breakfast prior to a task with high cognitive demand will also promote cognitive performance.

Caffeine: 1–3mg thirty to sixty minutes prior to performance of a complex cognitive task can improve cognitive performance. Caffeine will improve alertness, and may improve reaction time and accuracy of tasks. However, taking too much caffeine can lead to a decrement in performance.

Fruit and vegetables: Long-term intakes of fruit and vegetables seem to be related to improved cognitive performance. Cruciferous vegetables in particular appear to have positive effects on brain function when consumed over a long period of time.

Silver

Branched-chain amino acids: May reduce the production of serotonin in the brain, particularly when under significant physical fatigue.

Creatine: Creatine is a major fuel source for the brain, and in periods of high cognitive demand creatine concentration in the brain

NUTRITION AND THE BRAIN

can become depleted. Supplementation with doses as small as 5g prior to a cognitive task may improve performance.

Bronze

L-theanine: Particularly when taken in conjunction with caffeine can help to improve attention.

Polyphenols: A promising area of research where extracts of foods such as cocoa, which is a naturally high source of polyphenols, may improve cognitive function by improving blood flow to the brain.

Tyrosine: Supplementation with 100–300mg of tyrosine may improve cognitive performance. This may particularly be the case in periods of stress.

Omega 3 fatty acids: Omega 3 fatty acids, in particular docosahexaenoic acid (DHA), may influence brain function. Reaction time may be improved with 2.2g per day of omega 3 fatty acids for three weeks.

Further reading

Baker, L. B., Nuccio, R. P. & Jeukendrup, A. E. (2014). Acute effects of dietary constituents on motor skill and cognitive performance in athletes. *Nutrition Reviews*, 72(12), 790–802. doi:10.1111/nure.12157

Table 6.1 Example diet plan for Chapter 6.

Meal	Food
Breakfast	Large bowl of porridge made with semi-skimmed milk, with walnuts and raspberries. 125g pot of Greek yogurt 1 apple Cup of coffee
During exercise – skills-based session	750ml of 6% carbohydrate electrolyte drink with 1 isotonic carbohydrate gel
Post-exercise	1 apple, 1 handful of berries and 125g pot of quark cheese
Lunch	1 tin of tuna with a baked sweet potato and a mixed salad
Snack	2 slices of wholemeal bread with almond butter and a handful of berries
Dinner	1 chicken breast with broccoli, kale and carrots
Pre-bed snack	1 orange

Carbohydrate (g/kg body weight)	Protein (g/kg body weight)	Fat (g/kg body weight)
4	1.9	0.8

Bryan, J. (2008). Psychological effects of dietary components of tea: caffeine and L-theanine. *Nutrition Reviews*, 66(2), 82–90. doi:10.1111/j.1753-4887.2007.00011.x

Camfield, D. A., Stough, C., Farrimond, J. & Scholey, A. B. (2014). Acute effects of tea constituents L-theanine, caffeine, and epigallocatechin gallate on cognitive function and mood: a systematic review and meta-analysis. *Nutrition Reviews*, 72(8), 507–22. doi:10.1111/nure.12120

Kennedy, D. O. (2014). Polyphenols and the human brain: plant 'secondary metabolite' ecologic roles and endogenous signaling functions drive benefits. *Advances in Nutrition* (Bethesda, Md.), 5(5), 515–33.

CHAPTER 7

ENDURANCE EVENTS LASTING MORE THAN ONE HOUR

'Come on legs, lift the knees higher, go faster, why won't they go faster? If I can just get my legs to go a bit faster, lift the knees a touch higher, I can beat this guy, I can beat the pain. Concentrate, keep the focus. Don't give in, keep concentrating. No, I am not going to walk, no way. Well, maybe just for a short while, see if my legs can recover. No, I am not walking, I am keeping going. Keep concentrating, maybe I can if I just take a short walk. Oh, go on then let's walk. Now my mouth is dry, I would do anything for a pretzel. To taste the salt on my lips, to swill it down with a nice, ice-cold bottle of water. Maybe, if I'm lucky, if I can speed up again to the next food stop there will be salty pretzels, if I'm really lucky there will be some cola, flat preferably, but right now I would take anything. Ah, my mouth is so dry, I can't concentrate. Come on legs, keep moving, move faster, keep the knees up. Come on. How far to go now? If I speed up the end will come sooner, come on legs, move. Keep concentrating.'

This will be a pretty familiar narrative to those who have done endurance events: the confusion and pain at the end of an event lasting over an hour. Some of these events last for days on end, and these are the events upon which nutrition can have the biggest impact come race day.

To start to understand the nutritional needs of these long-distance endurance events we must first understand what causes fatigue. The clues are in the narrative. 'Come on legs, lift the knees higher' is a sign that the muscles cannot contract with the force that you might wish. 'Concentrate, keep the focus' is a sign that the brain and central nervous system are beginning to fatigue, to run out of fuel. 'Now my mouth is dry' indicates the body is becoming dehydrated. These are the three major reasons why an endurance athlete would become fatigued during a race, and in these three areas nutrition can play a role.

Let's start with muscle contraction. Muscle contracts by a series of filaments sliding and binding over each other. However, to do this energy is needed. As with all energy-needing processes in the body, this energy comes from the breakdown of adenosine triphosphate (ATP). However, there is not an endless supply of ATP available to the muscles to continually contract. To restock these limited energy stores, the body uses three main pathways. The first is an immediate source whereby the body uses creatine phosphate to resynthesize ATP. This system can help the muscle produce lots of force, but not for very long. The second is a system that can produce a reasonable amount of force, for a longer period of time, but doesn't need oxygen. The ATP from this process is derived from carbo-

ENDURANCE EVENTS LASTING MORE THAN ONE HOUR

hydrates, primarily glucose through the process of glycolysis, and leads to the formation of hydrogen ions, leading to an increase in pH and fatigue. Finally there is a third process, which requires oxygen, whereby through a number of processes, carbohydrate, fat and protein can be broken down to produce ATP. Fat is broken down through a process called beta oxidation, protein through a variety of processes such as the urea cycle and carbohydrate again through glycolysis. After these processes the end points enter a process called the Kreb's cycle and then the electron transport chain to produce ATP. The graph shows the relative force production and size of the potential energy production from each possible system.

During exercise, the contribution of protein to energy production is small and thought to be relatively insignificant. Fat and carbohydrate fight it out to produce ATP for the muscle to use. At a simple level, the lower the intensity of exercise, the more fat is used as a fuel; the higher the intensity of exercise, the more carbohydrate is used. The longer the event, the more fat as a fuel is also used, and the more aerobically trained the athlete, the more fat is used as a fuel.

We now know, therefore, that both fat and carbohydrate provide fuel for the muscles to produce the energy they need for exercise. So how big are the body's stores of these fuels? If we use calories as our measure of energy storage, an average male athlete

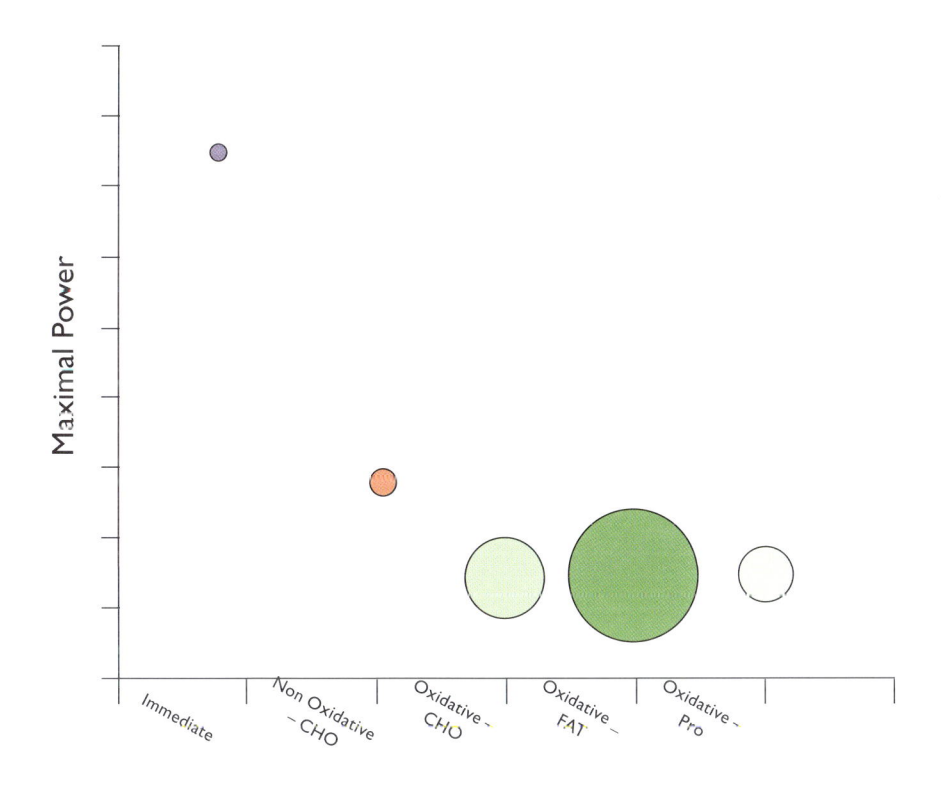

Relative energy storage and power for different energy systems in the muscle.

with an average body composition will store approximately 141,000 kcal of fat in his body. However, he will store only approximately 760 kcal of carbohydrate between the stores found in muscle glycogen and liver glycogen and a further 80 kcal found flowing around the body in blood. Carbohydrate stores are finite, therefore. Logically, once they are depleted fatigue sets in as the body cannot produce quite the same amount of force when burning fat as a fuel.

During endurance performance the body is continually burning a mixture of fat and carbohydrate. If we take the carbohydrate portion in isolation, as exercise duration continues there is a gradual reduction in muscle glycogen use and an increase in blood glucose use. Blood glucose is internally regulated by liver glycogen. The liver can synthesize glucose from other nutrients through a process called gluconeogenesis. However, this is not particularly efficient and eventually blood glucose will start to fall. Once this happens there is a reduction in the fuel supply to the muscle. This is the feeling of 'hitting the wall' if you are a runner, or 'hunger knock' or 'bonking' if you are a cyclist.

Another consequence of the reduction in blood glucose is a reduction in fuel to the brain. The brain is the master controller of all that occurs in the body. Therefore, a certain amount of central fatigue occurs. There is also some evidence of a signalling pathway between the concentration of muscle glycogen within the muscle and the brain.

'Now my mouth is dry' is the telling sign that it is time to drink. So how important is hydration in endurance performance? This has been debated in a lively way in sports science literature throughout the early part of the twenty-first century. If we went back 100 years the advice would be to avoid drinking during and around exercise as it would not be beneficial. Towards the end of the twentieth century research started to show a decrement in performance with dehydration.

The research as the twentieth century came to an end seemed to suggest that any amount of dehydration would be negative to performance. As I am sure everyone is aware, when you start to exercise you begin to sweat. This is a very individual response. We have all seen people in the gym who have a puddle around the treadmill, while the person next to them has only a light sheen of sweat on their brow. As we continue to exercise, the sweat continues to flow. The sweat we perspire takes fluid from plasma, the fluid component of the blood. Eventually this reduction in plasma volume leads to a compromise of cardiovascular function, in particular a decrease in cardiac output. This decreases the volume of blood which is able to flow to the skin, as there is a battle between skin and muscle for the blood that is flowing around. The muscle wants the fuel and the oxygen, while the skin wants the blood to be able to dissipate heat. The consequence of this is a decrease in heat dissipation and a subsequent rise in core temperature and the onset of fatigue.

However, this research, performed in a laboratory, has a major limitation. The laboratory misses one key aspect that real-world performance allows: wind speed. Imagine going out on your bike. Even if there is no wind you can feel the cooling effect of the air rushing past you. Go on a long descent and you can really feel it. Even at common running speeds, 10–20km per hour, there is a significant cooling effect of the air flowing past your skin. In laboratory-based studies, when wind speed has been matched with the effort and speed the athlete is undertaking, the effect of sweat loss is significantly reduced.

The ambient air temperature can also have an effect on performance. As temperature increases, so does sweat rate as a need to dissipate heat, therefore exacerbating the effects of fluid loss on cardiovascular function. A secondary effect of this increase in core body temperature is a change in fuel metabolism. An increase in core body temperature sees a switch to carbohydrate as a fuel away from fat metabolism. For prolonged events this could have a secondary effect on performance by increasing the rate of muscle glycogen usage and bringing into play another mechanism of fatigue.

However, it is not helpful to say that a particular degree of dehydration should be maintained. A recent meta-analysis on hydration and endurance performance has shown that starting exercise with greater than a 3 per cent loss of body water can decrease endurance performance. However, during time trials in outdoor conditions there is no evidence of a decrease in exercise performance with dehydration levels up to a 4 per cent body water loss. There are also a number of field-based studies, particularly in runners, which show that those who lose the most weight during races are those who run the quickest times.

So what does this mean? It seems that small to moderate levels of dehydration have a limited effect on performance. The ambient temperature will have an effect, with higher temperatures leading to a smaller threshold of dehydration. It is likely that the exact amount of dehydration that can be tolerated will be individual. The earlier laboratory studies give an example of an extreme situation where thermoregulation and cardiovascular function are compromised. It is likely that this

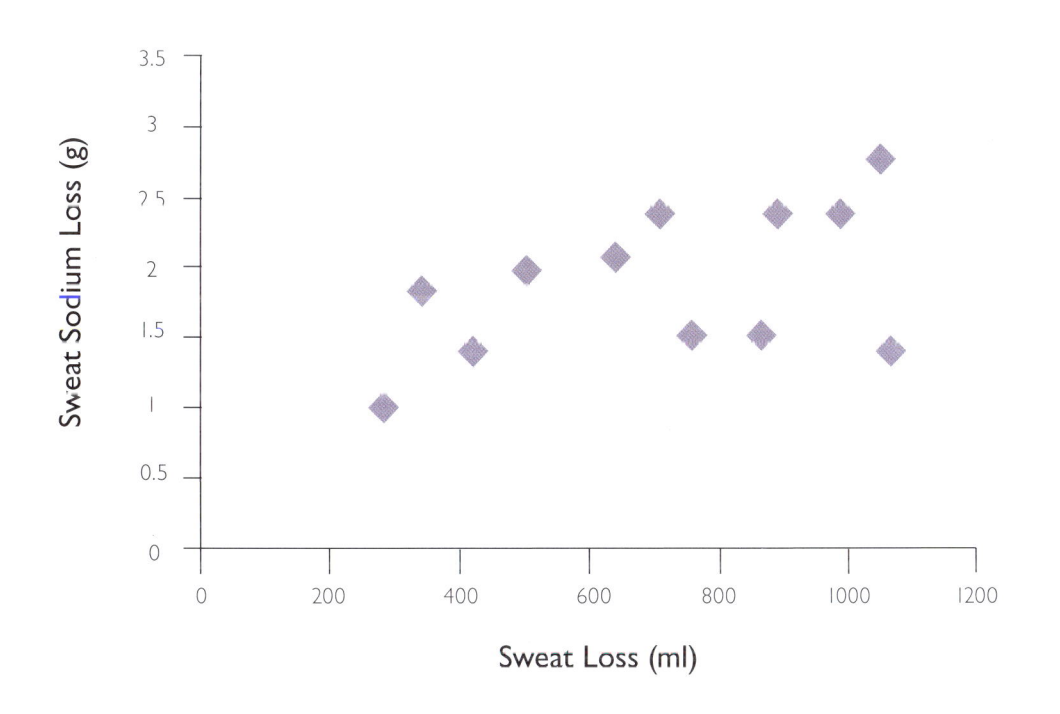

Sweat sodium and total sweat volume lost during a given training session in individual athletes.

will only occur in real-world situations in the most extreme and prolonged environments and events.

It certainly seems to make sense to begin a race hydrated. Without access to machines such as an osmometer, which can give a more accurate measure of hydration status, keeping an eye on urine colour leading into a race is a simple way to maintain hydration. If you are going to the toilet at regular intervals and your urine is lemonade-coloured, then you are hydrated. If your toilet trips are infrequent, and when you do go your urine is apple juice-coloured, you need to drink more. It should also be noted that there is large individual variation in the amount of fluid and sodium lost by athletes. This is illustrated in the graph which shows unpublished data of the variation in sweat loss and sweat sodium concentration for individual athletes performing the same training session.

All three major causes of fatigue during endurance exercise – a reduction in muscle contraction, cognitive fatigue and dehydration – can be influenced by nutrient intake around the race. Firstly, we will start with what you can do in the days leading up to the race to increase the size of your fuel tank. Secondly, we will look at what you can do during the race to maintain blood glucose and hydration. Finally, we will look at other ergogenic aids that might be useful during endurance performance.

Pre-race

Nutritional preparation for an endurance event starts days before the event itself begins. Your taper into the race will begin as you aim for a physical peak. What you eat and drink can have an effect on subsequent performance. The most well-known strategy is carbohydrate loading. We have all seen the pasta parties leading into races such as the London Marathon or an Ironman, where athletes are encouraged to eat as much carbohydrate as possible. Carbohydrate loading is as simple as it sounds. It is increasing the amount of carbohydrate an athlete consumes in order to increase muscle glycogen concentration.

The history of carbohydrate loading as a strategy to enhance endurance performance begins in the 1960s with the advent of the muscle biopsy technique and its use in exercise physiology. For the first time scientists could take a look at what happens within the muscle during exercise. In a series of neat studies performed in the laboratories of the legendary Scandinavian scientists Jonas Bergstrom and Eric Hultman, the relationship between muscle glycogen and fatigue was proven. As muscle glycogen concentration decreased so did performance, and a significant decrease in muscle glycogen concentration often coincided with fatigue.

Once the relationship between muscle glycogen and fatigue was established, the next logical step was to investigate whether increasing muscle glycogen concentration within the muscle led to a further delay in fatigue. The Scandinavians conducted studies where participants had three or four days of hard training with limited carbohydrate being consumed in their diet to decrease muscle glycogen concentration. Subsequent to this either a very high carbohydrate intake with limited training was undertaken, or a continuation of a low-carbohydrate diet. Unsurprisingly the carbohydrate loading group began exercise with a higher muscle glycogen concentration, and subsequently were able to exercise to fatigue for a longer period of time. Thus, the traditional carbohydrate loading protocol of a depletion phase, followed by a loading period, was born. This approach was taken into practice, and is still being used fifty years later.

ENDURANCE EVENTS LASTING MORE THAN ONE HOUR

Hard training for three days, coupled with a low carbohydrate intake, within one week of trying to hit peak performance does not seem optimal, and is in contrast to some tapering techniques. This approach will leave an athlete feeling tired, moody and at a greater risk of illness, none of which are conducive to peak performance. Further research in the 1980s, followed up in both the 1990s and 2000s, has shown that there does not need to be a 'depletion' phase to increase muscle glycogen concentration – rather, an approach to loading involving an increase in carbohydrate consumption to 8–12g per kg of body weight for two or three days prior to competition.

As with most things in life, there is always a flipside. While carbohydrate loading can delay fatigue in events lasting longer than ninety minutes, the approach is to delay the point where fatigue occurs, rather than increasing initial speed. If the event is longer than ninety minutes and of a high intensity, such as a triathlon or marathon, carbohydrate loading will improve performance. The carbohydrate loading protocol also leads to significant increase in body weight, as muscle glycogen is stored in the muscle bound to water. This can lead to an athlete feeling 'heavy'. An increased risk of gastrointestinal distress is also present, particularly as carbohydrates tend to come with fibre. Where possible, simple carbohydrates should be consumed.

A final consideration is the natural diet of an athlete. Many endurance athletes will naturally have a high-carbohydrate diet, consuming somewhere in the region of 8g of carbohydrate per kg of body weight. In this case the need to make a change to the diet is limited as athletes will taper into a race. This will naturally lead to a gap between carbohydrate intake and need, leading to an increase in muscle glycogen concentration.

Pre-event meal

'So, muscle glycogen is topped up. The morning alarm goes off. It's race day. Let's get ready to go race. Entering the kitchen or hotel breakfast service, what should I have? It's a tough choice, I will see what they've got. There's always something I can eat.'

In my experience the above approach is common to the pre-event meal, particularly the comment about seeing what's available in the hotel breakfast area. Yet the pre-event meal will have an effect on performance, both physiologically and psychologically. An athlete can control this meal.

Much research has been undertaken on pre-exercise carbohydrate intake and its effect on endurance performance. It clearly shows that ingesting 200–300g of low glycaemic index carbohydrates, three to four hours prior to exercise, improves performance compared to consuming nothing. Easier said

Table 7.1 Pros and cons of carbohydrate loading.

Pros	Cons
• Increases muscle glycogen concentration • May delay fatigue during long-duration events	• May not influence shorter distances • Difficult for females to do • May feel bloated • Increases risk of GI issues • Increases fibre intake • May lead to weight gain

ENDURANCE EVENTS LASTING MORE THAN ONE HOUR

> **GENDER DIFFERENCES IN CARBOHYDRATE LOADING**
>
> In 1995 research published from the research group of Mark Tarnopolsky from McMaster University in Canada suggested that there were gender differences in the ability to increase carbohydrate intake in order to increase muscle glycogen and therefore 'carbohydrate load'. Over a four-day period male and female runners were asked to increase the carbohydrate content of their diet from 55 per cent to 75 per cent of total energy intake. The results showed interesting differences in the ability of males and females to increase their muscle glycogen stores. The male runners increased their muscle glycogen content by 41 per cent over the four-day period. The females on the other hand showed no increase in muscle glycogen content.
>
> However, as carbohydrate was increased as a percentage of total energy intake, there were differences in total carbohydrate intake. The female participants consumed 6.4g per kg of body weight, whereas the males consumed 8.2g per kg of body weight.
>
> The same research group followed this up with a further study comparing male and female endurance athletes. This time there were three different conditions. One of them was just the habitual diet for four days, a second trial again increased carbohydrate intake to 75 per cent of total energy expenditure, and a third trial increased total energy intake by 34 per cent, and kept carbohydrate intake at 75 per cent.
>
> The male athletes once again increased muscle glycogen content in response to only increasing carbohydrate intake, whereas the females showed no increase. However, again total carbohydrate intake was different between the two genders, the females only consuming 6.4g per kg of body weight, and the males 7.9g per kg of body weight.
>
> With the extra energy in the third trial came significant amounts of extra carbohydrate. The males consumed 10.5g per kg of body weight, and the females 8.8g per kg of body weight per day. The female athletes were now able to increase muscle glycogen content, and the males showed a trend towards a further increase in muscle glycogen content.
>
> The gender differences in carbohydrate loading when expressed as a percentage of total energy expenditure are a function of different energy intakes. In both male and female athletes there seems to be a need to increase carbohydrate intake above 8g per kg of body weight to increase the glycogen content of muscle.

than done. Athletes are normally nervous and time-poor prior to an event, and taking this approach is not always easy.

What is less known is that fat and protein intake also improve performance compared to consuming nothing. Although this is not very well researched, it does seem to suggest that having something will improve performance. There is very little research investigating the effects of mixed meals on endurance performance. For instance, mixing protein with a carbohydrate-based meal will naturally decrease the glycaemic index of the meal. Athletes are often advised to avoid protein and fat in order to reduce gastrointestinal distress, with only anecdotal evidence to back this up.

So what should an athlete consume prior to exercise? This is dependent on the duration of the event, the type of exercise undertaken, the time of day of the event and the athlete's history of gastrointestinal distress. The decision tree here helps outline the decisions that need to be made.

ENDURANCE EVENTS LASTING MORE THAN ONE HOUR

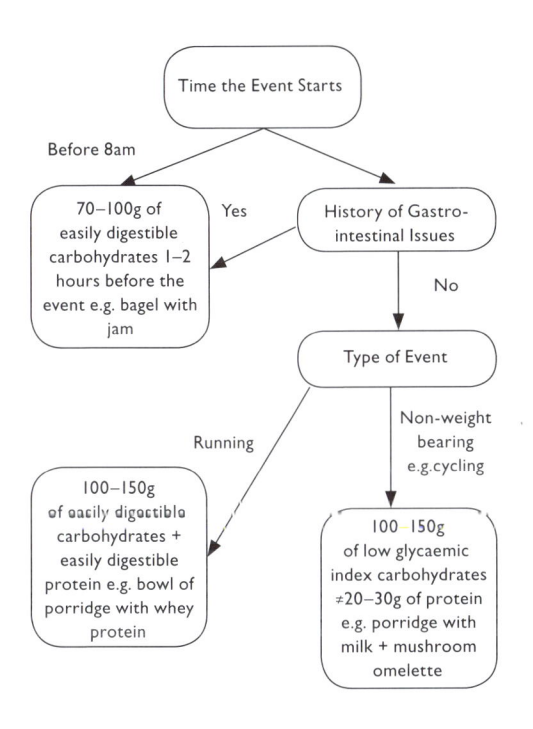

Decision tree for pre-event meal choice.

- Time the Event Starts
  - Before 8am → 70–100g of easily digestible carbohydrates 1–2 hours before the event e.g. bagel with jam
  - History of Gastro-intestinal Issues
    - Yes → 70–100g of easily digestible carbohydrates 1–2 hours before the event e.g. bagel with jam
    - No → Type of Event
      - Running → 100–150g of easily digestible carbohydrates + easily digestible protein e.g. bowl of porridge with whey protein
      - Non-weight bearing e.g. cycling → 100–150g of low glycaemic index carbohydrates ≠20–30g of protein e.g. porridge with milk + mushroom omelette

We already know that starting an endurance event in a dehydrated state will not lead to optimal performance. If urine colour is similar to apple juice, action needs to be taken and fluids consumed to restore hydration. It is advisable that fluid is consumed with the pre-event meal, and followed up with fluid into the race. The exact amount is individual in nature.

One option to consider is hyper-hydration. There is some evidence that this can improve performance. It essentially means loading up on fluid in the pre-race period, using sodium to retain the fluid. It will need specialist advice, though, as the sodium intake needed to do this is significantly above the recommended amount for healthy adults.

Gastrointestinal distress

You feel that first gurgle in your stomach, then all of a sudden a cramp occurs. Keep going, it

---

RESEARCH FOCUS

Sodium hyper-hydration and performance in the heat (Sims et al., 2007)

Sims and colleagues recruited eight endurance-trained athletes and got them to perform two runs to exhaustion at 70 per cent of VO_2 max in 32°C heat and 50 per cent humidity. On one occasion, 105 minutes prior to the start of the run, they started to consume approximately 750ml of a low-sodium drink which only contained 10 mmol/l of sodium. On a second occasion they consumed a drink containing 164 mmol/l of sodium. This is a similar concentration of sodium to that found in a saline drip used in hospitals. In order for this drink to be absorbed with such a high sodium content, a mixture of trisodium citrate and sodium chloride was used.

Ingesting the high-sodium drink led to a 4.5 per cent increase in plasma volume, whereas the low-sodium drink failed to increase plasma volume. During exercise the high-sodium drink led to a lower core temperature, heart rate and perceived exertion. There was also a slower increase in plasma osmolality with the high-sodium drink. In seven of the eight participants time to exhaustion was increased with the high-sodium drink compared to the low-sodium drink, with a range of performance improvements in those seven athletes from 5 per cent to 42 per cent. Improvements in time to exhaustion were strongly correlated with increases in plasma volume prior to the run.

ENDURANCE EVENTS LASTING MORE THAN ONE HOUR

will pass. Then another cramp comes, then another. All of a sudden you're holding out for the next bush you can hide behind. The cramps are excruciating. You have to walk. It's time to take on some more fuel. You can't do that as your stomach has screwed itself into a ball.

This situation is fairly common in people taking part in endurance events, running in particular, with reports of up to 70 per cent of individuals in endurance events suffering from feelings of stomach cramps or an urge to go to the toilet. These effects can significantly hinder performance, and in the worst cases can lead to significant complications. The cramps are generally caused by one or a combination of the following three factors:

- Physiological strain in the form of a reduction of blood flow to the intestine.
- Physical movement of the stomach and intestine, particularly in running events.
- Nutritional factors, such as fat, protein and fibre.

During races the body releases adrenaline. Adrenaline binds to receptors in the small intestine, leading to a reduction in blood flow to the stomach and intestine and a redirection of this blood flow to the working muscles. This reduction of blood flow, or ischemia, can lead to a reduction in oxygen and nutrients flowing to the intestine, making the smooth muscle of the intestine less efficient and more likely to cramp. Ischemia can also lead to feelings of nausea and diarrhoea. Damage to the intestine can also occur, leading to an increase in gut permeability. This increase in permeability leads to a cascade of events, resulting in an inflammatory response and fatigue.

The mechanical action of running can cause a jostling of the stomach and intestine, which itself can cause gastrointestinal distress. Lower abdominal pain and symptoms are more common in runners, and upper abdominal symptoms more so in cyclists due to the position of the body on the bike. There is very little that can be done to prevent these symptoms apart from training.

The final area is nutritional causes of gastrointestinal distress. While correlative in nature, there is evidence of a relationship between intake of fat, protein, fibre and dairy foods and the incidence of gastrointestinal symptoms. During exercise the intake of highly concentrated liquids containing carbohydrates, those with an osmolality of greater than 500 mOsm per litre, causes the greatest risk.

Athletes with a history of gastrointestinal distress have the greatest risk of another occurrence of gastrointestinal problems.

Table. 7.2 Common gastrointestinal symptoms during exercise.

Stomach Complaints	Stomach cramps Belching Nausea, including vomiting
Intestinal Complaints	Intestinal cramps Stitch Diarrhoea Bleeding in stools

Therefore, if you suffer from symptoms of gastrointestinal distress, the following should help reduce the incidence of symptoms:

- Begin exercise hydrated – dehydration will increase the risk of gastrointestinal problems.
- Train with the drinks, gels and other foods you intend to use during exercise to help your gut adapt to the demands you will place upon it.
- For one to three days prior to the race, decrease foods that are more likely to cause irritation to the intestine and lead to gastrointestinal distress.
- Avoid aspirin and ibuprofen – these have been shown to reduce absorption of nutrients from the gut and can lead to an increased risk of gastrointestinal symptoms.
- More novel and experimental solutions involve supplementing with probiotics and colostrum to increase gastrointestinal health, along with pre-exercise supplementation of beetroot juice or L-citrulline to increase blood flow to the small intestine. These solutions should be tried in conjunction with an expert to show you the best way to use the supplements.

In-event fuelling

Once the race begins, feeding can start. The most important nutrient to consider is carbohydrate, and in its simplest form – sugar. The first scientific studies on ingesting carbohydrate, and specifically sugar, were in the early 1920s. In a series of applied trials researchers investigated the effects of sugar ingestion – or not – during the Boston Marathon. There seemed to be a trend that those who consumed sugar during the race ran faster. From here, things seem to go quiet for almost sixty years. While there was some interest in ingesting carbohydrate and exercise performance in the 1960s and 1970s, it was in the 1980s that things really started to take off through the lab of Professor Eddie Coyle at the University of Texas. Professor Coyle led a team of researchers to conduct a series of studies using a test called a 'time to exhaustion' protocol. The protocols were first developed for use in animal research. They employ a method of exercising individuals at a set intensity until they can no longer continue at that intensity and exhaustion is reached. While debate continues over the validity of these tests as a measure of performance due to the lack of a pacing component, they are quite useful when looking at mechanisms. Using these protocols, Professor Coyle and his team showed that when you take on board simple sugars during endurance exercise, compared to water, exhaustion occurs at a time point 17 per cent further on than water alone. Throughout these studies it was shown that exhaustion occurs at the point blood sugar begins to decrease, in both conditions. However, consuming sugar delayed the fall in blood sugar compared to water. There is some evidence, particularly in running exercise, that consuming carbohydrate during exercise also spares muscle glycogen. However, this is less conclusive. There is also evidence that ingesting carbohydrate during exercise maintains cognitive function more effectively than water.

So what type, and what amount, of carbohydrate can maximize exercise performance? This was a question Professor Asker Jeukendrup and his team at the University of Birmingham set out to investigate in the late 1990s and early 2000s. As a matter of disclosure I should point out that I was a member of this team and conducted some of the later work we will talk about. Professor Jeukendrup and team set out to feed the simplest of sugars –

ENDURANCE EVENTS LASTING MORE THAN ONE HOUR

glucose – at a rate of 1g/min during two hours of exercise. They then used the latest stable isotope technology to analyse how much of the glucose was burnt by the body. It turns out that it was in the region of 0.8–1g/min. So they fed more glucose at a rate of 1.8g/min. However, the body still only burnt 0.8–1g/min. Maybe a limit had been found? Where could that limit be? Earlier studies had shown that if you infuse glucose through a saline drip your muscles can pretty much burn the glucose at whatever rate it was infused. So by logical deduction the intestine should be the limiting factor of carbohydrate oxidation by muscles.

Basic gut physiology tells us that there are two predominant transporters of sugar across the intestine: sodium glucose transporter 1 (SGLT-1), which transports sugars such as glucose and galactose (found in honey); and glucose transporter 5 (GLUT5), which transports fructose (a fruit-based sugar). What would happen if we fed two different types of sugar, one of which is transported through SGLT-1 and another through GLUT5?, asked the authors. What they found was that they could feed high rates of carbohydrate when a mixture of glucose and fructose was combined in a 2:1 ratio compared to the same rate of glucose alone and this led to an increase in oxidation of these sugars by up to 50 per cent. They also managed to show that this combination of sugars also increased the absorption of water through the intestine.

So what, you might ask? Does this make me go faster? This was a question I set out to answer in my PhD studies. We designed a cycling-based protocol whereby subjects entered the laboratory at 7am with no breakfast. They then cycled for two hours at a moderate intensity, and followed this up with a time trial that lasted approximately one hour. Using this final time trial as our

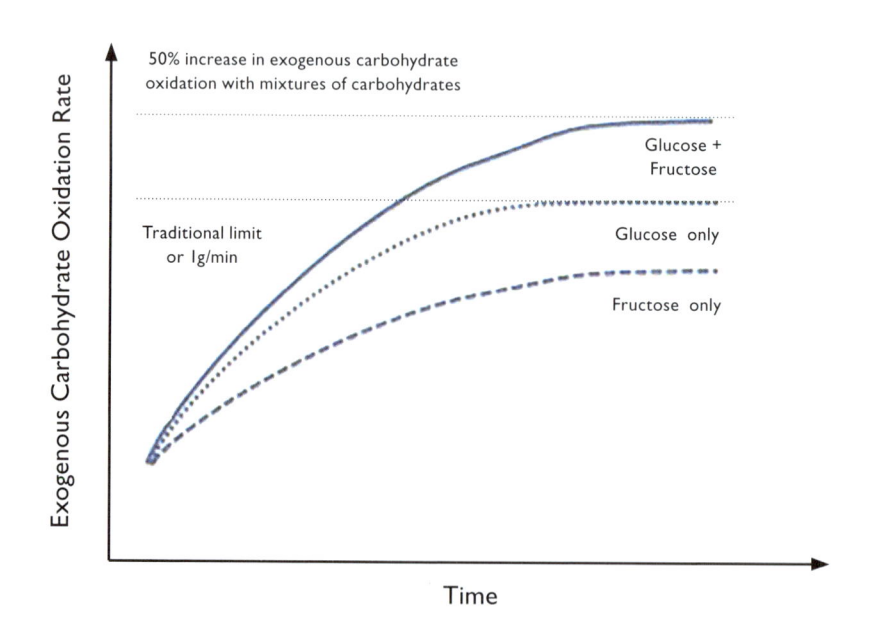

A combination of glucose and fructose increases exogenous carbohydrate oxidation.

ENDURANCE EVENTS LASTING MORE THAN ONE HOUR

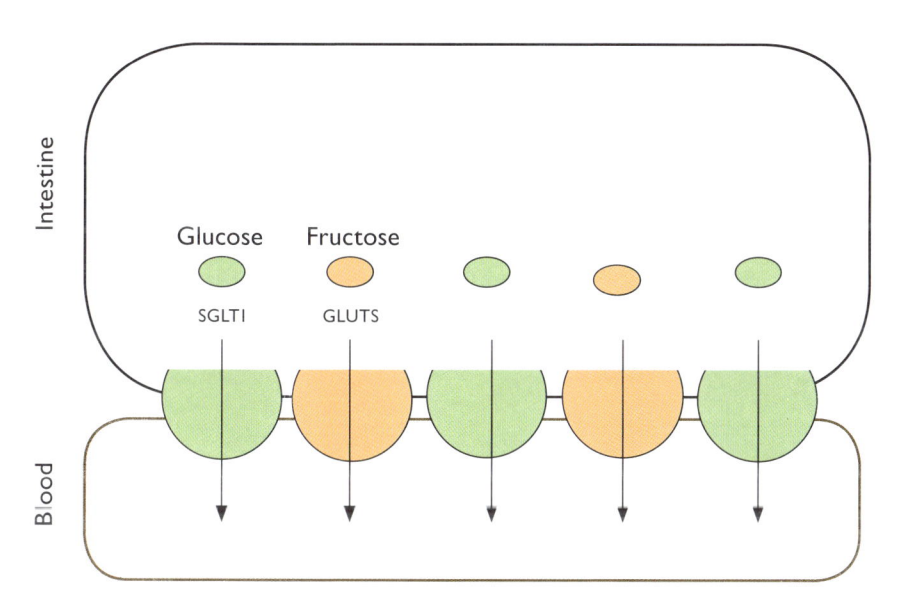

Simplified schematic of how the addition of fructose increases intestinal absorption of carbohydrate by using different absorption pathways other than glucose.

performance marker, we discovered that consuming glucose at a rate of 1.8g/min throughout the whole trial increased performance by 8 per cent compared to a flavoured placebo. When the glucose and fructose mixture was consumed there was an 8 per cent improvement in performance compared to glucose alone, and a whopping 16 per cent over the placebo condition. Fortunately, other studies have shown similar patterns since this work was published. It should be noted that it is unlikely that everyone will get such big effects from consuming carbohydrate in this way. This was an artificial, laboratory-based condition. However, it is clear that for endurance performance a mixture of glucose and fructose is the optimal combination of sugar. There also seems to be a sweet spot of consumption around about 70–80g/min of carbohydrate to maximize performance.

As we found out earlier in this chapter, there is contention about the role of fluid intake during endurance events and the effect this has on performance. From laboratory-based studies, consuming adequate fluids to match fluid losses improves performance, as against *ad libitum* drinking. However, when *ad libitum* or drinking to thirst is used in real-world situations, there does not seem to be an added benefit compared to matching fluid losses. These data suggest that the body has its own regulatory mechanisms to allow athletes to drink to regulate fluid intake.

In principle the idea of drinking to thirst seems a solid suggestion. However, in practice it is not as simple as it first seems due to the demands of the event. In events like road cycling fluid intake is relatively simple as bottles can easily be carried on the bike. However, for events such as marathon running, there are limited opportunities for fluid intake. Therefore, a plan needs to be devised to allow fluid to be drunk according to thirst.

The composition of fluid also needs to be

ENDURANCE EVENTS LASTING MORE THAN ONE HOUR

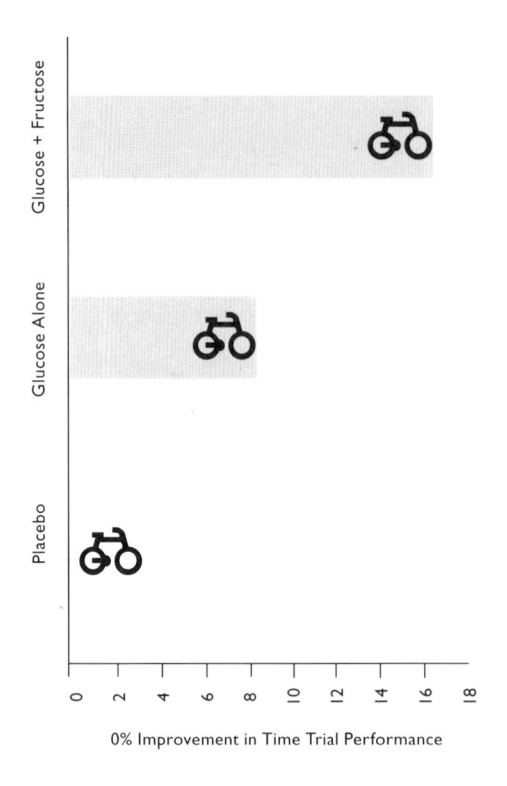

Improvement in cycling time-trial performance with different carbohydrate mixtures (adapted from Currell et al., 2008).

considered as the fluid will most likely provide a source of carbohydrate, too. There is lots of information about the tonicity of drink-taking during exercise, with isotonic claiming to be the ideal. This means the solid component of the fluid is similar to that found in the body. However, there is very little evidence that the tonicity of the drink you consume makes that much difference to performance.

In order to be absorbed, fluid must first pass through the stomach. The energy density of the drink, or amount of carbohydrate, usually affects this process. The fluid is then absorbed primarily in the small intestine, through a process of osmosis. Therefore, there is some advantage to ensuring the osmotic gradient across the intestine is in favour of flow into the bloodstream. In reality this is difficult to control in a real-world situation.

Fluid is also absorbed through the process of glucose absorption. For every molecule of glucose actively absorbed within the intestine, 300 molecules of water pass through with it. There are also potential mechanisms by which fluid can pass with fructose absorption. Research suggests that not only is a carbohydrate drink consisting of glucose and fructose the most effective way to get sugar into the bloodstream, it is also the most effective way of absorbing fluid.

Sweat sodium losses can be significant, therefore sodium is often added to sports drinks to offset this and enhance absorption of fluid through the intestine. Sodium in sports drinks will also help to maintain extra cellular volume. There is very little evidence that sodium intake enhances performance during exercise. However, there is strong anecdotal evidence from endurance athletes that salt intake during prolonged exercise is important. This seems particularly to be the case for 'salty' sweaters. The simplest way to see if you are a salty sweater is to check out your training kit after training. It is likely to be covered in a white powder, suggesting the presence of significant amounts of salt. Typically, sports drinks will contain 20–30 mmol per litre of salt. For those who sweat more, the concentration of salt could be increased to 30–50 mmol/l to try to offset some of the sweat sodium losses.

A final factor in choosing fluid replacement during exercise is taste. It is likely that significant amounts of fluid will be consumed in an endurance race. Choosing a drink that you like the taste of is key. Also, be aware that taste changes as fatigue sets in, and it is very easy for flavour fatigue to set in during endurance events.

Overdrinking is also a concern in endurance events. It can lead to a condition termed hyponatraemia – essentially a low plasma sodium concentration. Hyponatraemia is a serious condition with a long list of consequences, the worst of which is death. There are likely to be many complications leading to this dangerous state. Those at greatest risk are slower, heavier athletes who have a longer period of time to consume fluids during an event. What is clear from this area of research is that athletes should not drink significant amounts of fluid such as they increase their body weight. There are reported cases in endurance events such as marathons and Ironman races of athletes increasing their body weight by up to 8 per cent. When sweat losses are taken into account athletes must be consuming significant volumes of fluid for this to occur. However, by drinking to thirst the risk of hyponatraemia can be reduced.

Caffeine

Caffeine is one of the most used and socially acceptable drugs in the world. It is all around us. Coffee is what we most associate with caffeine, but it can be found in tea, drinks such as cola, and chocolate, to name but a few. Alongside this, raw caffeine can be purchased in any pharmacy, and more and more supplements seem to contain caffeine. For many years caffeine was on the WADA list of prohibited substances and therefore not able to be used in sporting events. All that changed in 2004, when the rules were altered and caffeine was permitted.

Caffeine clearly improves performance. It is one of the few supplements that improves performance across events and disciplines. Research has shown that it can improve performance of short-duration events such as weight-lifting, through to ultra-endurance events. Of course many people use caffeine to improve their performance at work, or even their dancing performance in a nightclub.

So how does caffeine work? In terms of endurance events, there are a number of ways. One of the most common suggested mechanisms is through an increase in fat metabolism and sparing of muscle glycogen. Despite this being a common suggestion and caffeine even being used to help weight loss, the latest research would suggest that there is no effect of caffeine on fat metabolism. There are some potential mechanisms where caffeine interacts directly with the muscle to influence muscle function, but is unlikely to affect endurance performance.

Most promising is the interaction that caffeine has with adenosine receptors in the brain. Interaction with these receptors leads to a stimulation of the central nervous system function. Subsequent to this, there is a likely decrease in perceptions of pain and ratings of perceived exertion. This suppression of pain and reduction in perception of effort leads to an improvement in performance.

Many historical studies have used high doses of caffeine prior to an event to improve endurance performance. These high doses of 6mg per kg of body weight clearly lead to performance improvement. However, more recent studies have shown that doses in the region of 1–3mg per kg of body weight can also lead to performance improvement.

Generally it is advisable to coincide the intake of caffeine with peak caffeine concentrations within the blood. This occurs on average sixty minutes after consumption of the caffeine dose. The effects of caffeine appear to last for up to six hours after ingestion in those who are unaccustomed to it. In those who habitually consume caffeine, the effect lasts for up to three hours. Those who habitually consume it do not need to refrain from caffeine intake in the lead-up to a race to gain an effect. Caffeine has been shown to be equally effective in habitual users as well as non-users.

More recent studies have compared different sources of caffeine and their effect on endurance performance. Coffee, supplied at an identical dose of caffeine, is just as effective as caffeine tablets. Caffeine gum is also an effective method of consuming caffeine, but must be taken closer to the start of an event for it to be effective.

Surprisingly little research has been undertaken on the effect of caffeine during exercise, despite a number of products available containing caffeine that are aimed at mid-race consumption. One of the few studies to do so, from the Australian Institute of Sport, showed an approximately 3 per cent improvement in performance when repeated doses were given of 1mg per kg of body weight throughout two hours of exercise, with a time trial following. This suggests that there is a performance effect of consuming caffeine during an endurance event such as a marathon or a triathlon. Athletes should aim for 50–100mg of caffeine per hour of exercise to maximize performance.

There are possible side effects to using caffeine during exercise. One of them is the potential to cause dehydration, though there is no evidence that caffeine or coffee cause dehydration. However, those who have a known heart condition should consult their doctor prior to using caffeine due to the increase in heart rate and blood pressure that can be seen with caffeine intake.

A final consideration is the importance of sleep to an athlete's performance. Caffeine will disrupt normal sleep cycles, and if taken too late in the day can lead to disrupted sleep. In contrast to this, caffeine is likely to be even more effective in conditions of sleep deprivation. Certainly those early-morning starts that many endurance races have could be offset by caffeine use.

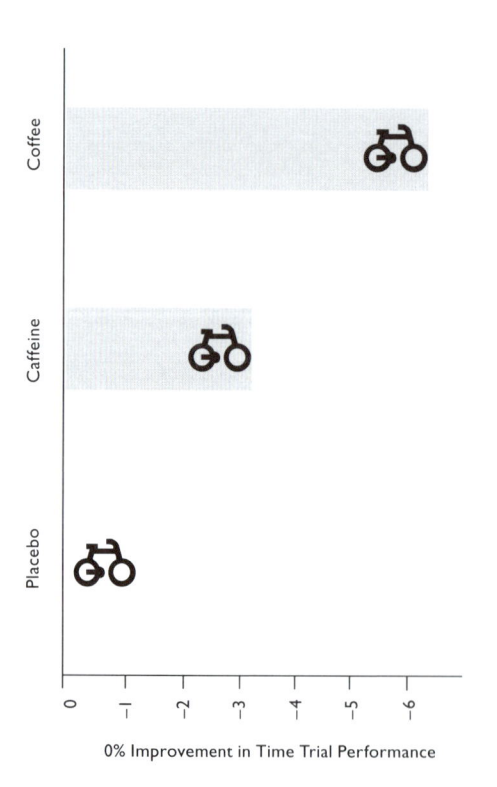

Per cent change in time-trial performance with caffeine and coffee compared to placebo (Hodgson et al., 2013).

Nitrates

Finally we are left with the new kid on the block – beetroot. Unbelievably, the humble beetroot leads to an improvement in performance. It is all down to a small component of the beetroot, called nitrate.

The nitrate we find in our diet, of which beetroot is just one source, is absorbed through the gut, from where it is returned to the mouth to be broken down into nitrite. Nitrite is then reabsorbed and through a biochemical process is broken down to nitric oxide. Nitric oxide is a potent modulator of many physiological processes within the body.

These processes include a number that lead to an improvement in exercise performance. An increase in nitric oxide will lead to an increase in blood flow to the muscle, a decrease in the oxygen cost of a given exercise intensity, and will make the muscle more efficient at producing energy. All of these add up to a potential improvement in exercise performance.

It seems that chronic supplementation of dietary nitrates over three to six days of consuming 5–7 mmol per day will lead to an improvement in performance. Higher acute doses may also be effective, although the jury is still out on this. Dietary nitrate supplementation may be more effective in sub-elite athletes, as nitric oxide production is already upregulated in elite athletes. Alternatively, a higher dose may be needed to exhibit an increase in nitric oxide. At present data is not available to give an answer, and it is likely to be variable between athletes.

Heat

As ambient temperature increases, a greater challenge is put on the body to perform and cope with the exercise being undertaken. Exercise in the heat increases the thermoregulatory burden on the body, and in particular the cardiovascular system, which leads to challenges for brain function, ventilator function and muscle metabolism.

While exercising in the heat, core body temperature is raised due to the increase in environmental temperature and increases in metabolic heat production. This leads to an imbalance in the heat gain and release of the body towards a larger gain in heat. The consequence of this increased heat gain is fatigue, which is caused by a complex interplay of mechanisms both at the local level of the muscle and at the level of the brain.

Two aspects of nutritional preparation should be considered when it is necessary to exercise in the heat. The first is hydration status and fluid intake. During exercise in the heat athletes should begin exercise in a euhydrated state, and then consider fluid intake during exercise to minimize the negative performance effects of dehydration. See Chapter 5 for further information on fluid intake during exercise.

MONITORING HYDRATION STATUS

There are many devices available that will allow athletes to monitor their hydration status, normally by using a urine sample. Some of these, such as measuring urine osmolality or urine specific gravity, essentially measure how many solid molecules appear in the urine and give an idea of how concentrated the urine is.

However, there is a simple, cost-effective method which in research appears to be just as effective as using more expensive tools to monitor hydration status. Urine colour can give a very good indication of how hydrated an athlete is. If urine is pale in colour then the athlete is likely to be hydrated, whereas if urine is dark in colour then the athlete is more likely to be dehydrated.

Urine colour can be affected by food intake. A high intake of B vitamins can lead to urine becoming very yellow in colour, therefore making it hard to use urine as a hydration monitor. Intake of beetroot juice can turn urine red, again making it difficult to use urine to monitor hydration status.

The second area for nutritional preparation in the heat is the increased carbohy-

ENDURANCE EVENTS LASTING MORE THAN ONE HOUR

drate demands of exercise. The increase in core temperature leads to a shift in muscle metabolism towards using carbohydrate as a fuel, and in particular muscle glycogen. Therefore a period of increased carbohydrate intake prior to performance will be beneficial to performance.

Altitude

Some athletes need to compete at altitude. Even exposure to performance at moderate altitudes such as 1,000–2,000m can lead to a decrement in performance. Obviously, with an increase in altitude above sea level comes a decrease in the amount of oxygen available due to the decrease in barometric pressure, which leads to less oxygen for a given volume of air.

Maximal oxygen uptake begins to decrease at around 1,500m in most people, although there is some thought that the effect might start to occur at lower altitudes than this, particularly in well-trained athletes. Along with this decrease in maximal oxygen uptake is an increase in both heart rate and ventilation at rest and during exercise. There is an increase in blood pressure and increases in catecholamine secretion.

These changes in physiological function lead to a decrease in performance compared to sea-level performance, whether running a 800m race, repeated sprinting in a football match or running a marathon. The degree to which performance is impaired is very individual and seems to be linked to an individual's ability to defend arterial oxygen saturation.

One nutritional method which has been explored to defend arterial oxygen saturation is caffeine. Caffeine ingestion generally leads to an increase in ventilatory rate. Athletes who show a greater desaturation of oxygen in the blood generally have a lower ventilator drive and caffeine can be used to overcome this response.

Researchers from Indiana University in the USA took eight caffeine-naïve athletes who all desaturated considerably, and supplemented them with 8mg of caffeine per kg of body weight before a progressive exercise test to exhaustion. At lower levels of exercise intensity there was a greater oxygen saturation after caffeine ingestion, along with an increase in ventilator rates. As exercise reached maximal intensities this response didn't occur, probably because the exercise drive led to a greater response than the caffeine and a maximal mechanical threshold of ventilation was reached. However, this is a very high dose of caffeine, and while lower doses such as 3mg/kg of body weight have not been proven, they are more realistic and practical.

If there is a decrease in oxygen availability, what if we could provide an intervention that makes muscle more efficient at using oxygen? The humble beetroot seems able to do just that. Supplementation of beetroot juice prior to exercise reduces the oxygen of exercise. Could this work in hypoxia, too?

The research on the effects of beetroot juice, and its magic ingredient dietary nitrate, has been pioneered by Professor Andy Jones and his research group from the University of Exeter. The area of beetroot juice and exercise in hypoxia is no different. In the first of their studies nine healthy participants completed a leg-kicking exercise protocol until exhaustion in normal oxygen conditions and twice further with reduced oxygen concentrations in the air they were breathing. For one of these hypoxic conditions the participants drank 0.75l of beetroot juice, which contained 9.3 mmol of nitrate, or a beetroot juice placebo that contained no nitrate.

Interestingly, supplementing with beetroot juice prior to exercise in hypoxia prevented the decrease in performance usually seen compared to normal conditions, with many changes in the muscle suggesting fewer metabolic changes than usual. A further study using cycling exercise showed that during severe-intensity exercise, which took approximately three minutes to complete, there was a significant improvement in performance when beetroot juice was supplemented. In a follow-up study looking at how the muscle recovers after exercise in hypoxia, the research group were able to show that beetroot juice increases metabolic recovery of the muscle, and speeds up the rate at which ATP resynthesis occurs.

For more prolonged exercise a further challenge is a change in fuel use during exercise from fat to carbohydrate, and in particular an increase in blood glucose use as a fuel. This change is likely due to the decreased availability of oxygen to enter the muscle and therefore be used in aerobic metabolism processes. Along with this, the increase in blood glucose use as a fuel may be driven by the increased catecholamine release as a response to the altitude exposure.

The increased use of blood glucose can be a challenge as there is a finite ability for the body to maintain blood glucose during periods of high utilization. A reduction in blood glucose can lead to a decrease in performance. The simplest way to maintain blood glucose is to consume carbohydrates during exercise to maintain blood glucose. Consuming carbohydrates at a rate of 60–90g per hour would be optimal, with further explanation in Chapter 10 on the mechanisms of this effect.

As mentioned, a response to exercise at altitude is an increase in ventilatory rate. A consequence of this is an increase in total water expired during breathing. This makes it more difficult for an athlete to maintain hydration status, which should be monitored throughout exposures to altitude to help athletes maintain the correct level.

Summary

- Performance in endurance events is determined by the ability to continually resynthesize the necessary ATP stores within the muscle. These need to be continually replaced throughout the event.
- ATP is resynthesized through metabolic pathways that break down carbohydrate, fat and protein to produce ATP. Carbohydrate and fat are the predominant fuels used during exercise.
- As intensity increases, so does carbohydrate use. As duration increases, there is a shift in fuel use from carbohydrate to fat. Within the carbohydrate sources there is also a shift towards using more blood glucose as a fuel as exercise continues.
- Blood glucose is a finite store and needs to be maintained, otherwise fatigue occurs.
- Dehydration can also cause fatigue. However, it is potentially not as important as once thought. There is likely to be an individual set point beyond which dehydration negatively impacts on performance.
- Gastrointestinal issues are common in endurance events. They can be caused by the physiological strain of exercise, the physical movement of the stomach and intestine, or intake of nutrients such as fat, protein and fibre.
- Endurance athletes may have to compete in different environments: in the heat or at altitude.

ENDURANCE EVENTS LASTING MORE THAN ONE HOUR

Gold

Carbohydrate loading: Consuming 8g per kg of body weight the day before the race will increase muscle glycogen concentrations and delay the point at which fatigue occurs.

Pre-exercise carbohydrate intake: Consuming 2–3g per kg of body weight two to three hours prior to an endurance event will improve performance during the event. Where possible, carbohydrates with a low glycaemic index should be chosen.

Begin hydrated: Beginning an event hydrated should be promoted where possible. Monitor urine colour and output prior to events to ensure hydration. This is particularly key when performing in the heat.

Carbohydrate intake during exercise: Consuming 60–90g per hour of carbohydrates made up of either glucose or maltodextrin, with the addition of fructose in an 2:1 ratio, will improve endurance performance. Begin fuelling at the beginning of the event to maximize the effect.

Fluid intake during: Consuming fluid to thirst demands currently seems to provide the optimal way to maintain hydration during exercise. However, as fluids come with carbohydrates it is likely that there will need to be a plan in place to mix fluids and fuel.

Table 7.3 Example diet plan for Chapter 7.

Meal	Food
Breakfast	Large bowl of porridge made with semi-skimmed milk, with walnuts and raspberries 125g pot of Greek yogurt 1 apple 1 probiotic yogurt Cup of tea with milk
Snacks	2 bananas 1 isotonic carbohydrate gel and 750ml of 6% carbohydrate electrolyte drink
Snacks	1 bagel with jam
Lunch	1 tin of tuna with a baked sweet potato and a mixed salad
Snack	1 bagel with jam, 750ml of 6% carbohydrate drink
Snack	1 muffin with a handful of blueberries
Dinner	1 chicken breast with brown rice, broccoli, kale and carrots
Pre-bed snack	4 slices of malt loaf

Carbohydrate (g/kg body weight) 1.8	Protein (g/kg body weight) 2.1	Fat (g/kg body weight) 0.7

Caffeine: 1–3mg of caffeine taken thirty to ninety minutes prior to the event will improve performance. For prolonged events small doses of 50mg of caffeine every hour will help maintain performance throughout.

Silver
Nitrates: Consuming 5–7 mmol per day of nitrate for three to six days prior to the race will improve performance by improving efficiency of oxygen use. This may be particularly useful when competing at altitude.

Bronze
Hyperhydration: Using sodium to hyperhydrate prior to an event may improve performance, particularly in the heat.

Caffeine for altitude performance: There is some evidence that caffeine supplementation may offset some of the adverse ventilator events seen at altitude.

Further reading

Burke, L. M., Hawley, J. A, Wong, S. H. S. & Jeukendrup, A. E. (2011). Carbohydrates for training and competition. *Journal of Sports Sciences*, 29 Suppl 1(June 2011), S17–27. doi:10.1080/02640414.2011.585473

Cox, G. R., Desbrow, B., Montgomery, P. G., Anderson, M. E., Bruce, C. R., Macrides, T. A, Burke, L. M. (2002). Effect of different protocols of caffeine intake on metabolism and endurance performance. *Journal of Applied Physiology* (Bethesda, Md. : 1985), 93(3), 990–9. doi:10.1152/japplphysiol.00249.2002

Currell, K. & Jeukendrup, A. E. (2008). Superior endurance performance with ingestion of multiple transportable carbohydrates. *Medicine and Science in Sports and Exercise*, 40(2), 275–81. doi:10.1249/mss.0b013e31815adf19

Goulet, E. D. B. (2011). Effect of exercise-induced dehydration on time-trial exercise performance: a meta-analysis. *British Journal of Sports Medicine*, 45(14), 1149–56. doi:10.1136/bjsm.2010.077966

Stellingwerff, T. & Cox, G. R. (2014). Systematic review: Carbohydrate supplementation on exercise performance or capacity of varying durations. *Applied Physiology, Nutrition, and Metabolism = Physiologie Appliquée, Nutrition et Métabolisme*, 39(9), 998–1011. doi:10.1139/apnm-2014-0027

CHAPTER 8

EVENTS LASTING LESS THAN ONE HOUR AND WITH MULTIPLE ROUNDS

Many people in sport will have experienced that sting in the muscle, that metallic taste in the mouth or that screaming pain during short-term, high-intensity exercise. Many events shorter than an hour in duration are characterized by an increase of lactate in the blood. This is caused by an increase in the rate of glycolysis within the muscle to such an extent that pyruvate cannot be converted to acetyl-CoA for entry into the Kreb's cycle quickly enough. The lactate is then transported out of the muscle into the blood through transporters called monocarboxylic transporters (MCTs). Of course everyone knows that lactate causes fatigue. Or does it?

To explore this a little more let's go back to the discovery of lactate and lactic acid. Lactic acid gets its name from first being discovered in soured milk by the Swedish scientist Carl Wilhelm Scheele in 1780. While lactic acid was shown to be present in many organisms, its role in exercise in humans was not cemented until the classical research of the Nobel Prize-winning scientists Archibald V. Hill and Otto Meyerhoff in the 1920s. These eminent scientists showed that lactic acid was the end point of glycolysis, and in particular was increased when the rate of glycolysis exceeded that of oxidative metabolism or what would later become known as the Kreb's cycle (once it was fully discovered by another Nobel Prize-winning scientist, Hans Kreb).

Following on from these groundbreaking discoveries it was established that along with an increase in lactic acid came a decrease in both muscle and blood pH, with an almost perfect inverse correlation between increases in lactic acid and decreases in pH. Of course, a decrease in pH means a shift towards an acidic environment. Subsequently, a number of scientists showed that an acidic environment is one of the causes of fatigue in muscle. Thus the idea was born that lactic acid causes fatigue.

However, like many things born out of correlations and assumptions, lactic acid does not appear to cause fatigue at all. In fact the body cleverly produces lactate as an end point of glycolysis as an energy store, to be used by muscle or other organs as an energy source when needed.

However, an increase in lactate production does give us an indication that the metabolic process of glycolysis, which is the breakdown of glucose to produce energy, is in full swing. There are nine steps in glycolysis, which start with glucose-6-phosphate. To produce glucose-6-phosphate the muscle either breaks down glucose or muscle glycogen.

EVENTS LASTING LESS THAN ONE HOUR AND WITH MULTIPLE ROUNDS

Percentage of muscle glycogen depletion after exercise efforts of different durations and therefore intensities (adapted from Gollnick et al., 1974).

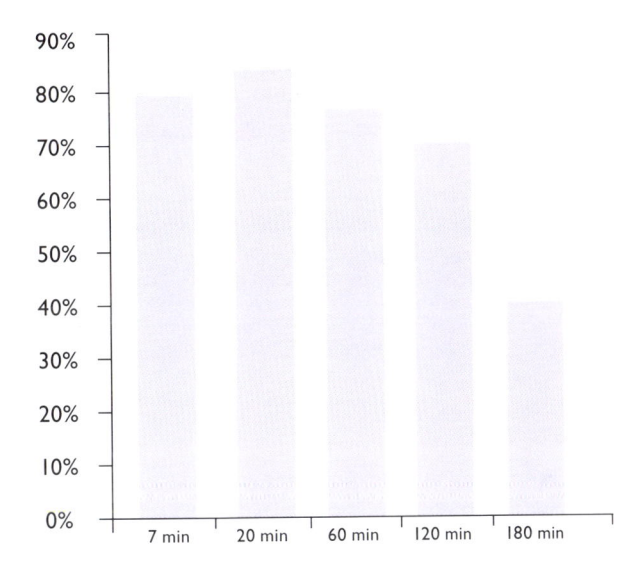

During this process of breaking down carbohydrate to produce energy, hydrogen ions are produced. Hydrogen ions drive the decrease in pH and are one of the causes of fatigue in high-intensity exercise. Glycolysis produces five hydrogen ions for each molecule of glucose-6-phosphate oxidized, and consumes two, leaving a net hydrogen ion production of three for every turn of glycolysis. When exercise intensity is low enough for this acid to be buffered and metabolized within the mitochondria of the muscle, there is no significant increase in pH. However, when exercise intensity increases, hydrogen ions keep being produced at a rate that cannot be matched by the muscles' inherent buffering systems and an increase in pH is seen. Fatigue ensues.

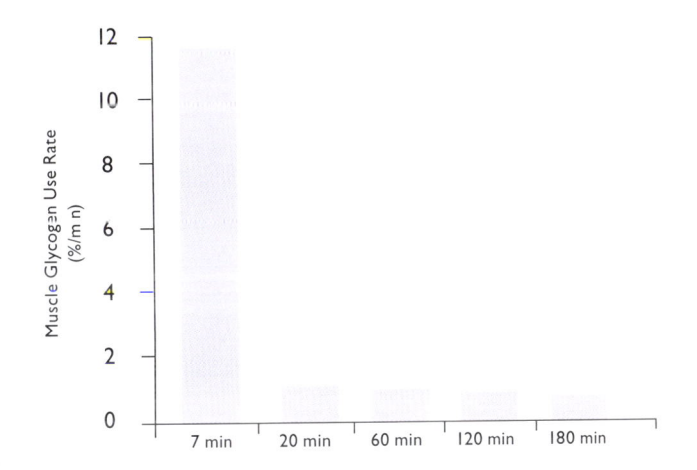

Rate of muscle glycogen utilization for events of differing duration (adapted from Gollnick et al., 1974).

EVENTS LASTING LESS THAN ONE HOUR AND WITH MULTIPLE ROUNDS

Nutritional buffers

The body has in-built systems that buffer the acid produced during high-intensity muscle contraction. These include proteins, peptides (short chains of amino acids) and amino acids themselves within the muscle, along with phosphates. Transporting hydrogen ions out of the muscle is important too (through MCTs), where hydrogen ions are primarily buffered by bicarbonates.

Nutritional intake can primarily affect two aspects. One is found within the muscle, in the form of the dipeptide carnosine. The second is by increasing the bicarbonate content of the blood. Let's start with carnosine.

Carnosine was first discovered by a Russian scientist called Vladimir Gulevich, and is pre-dominantly found in the skeletal muscle of mammals. In human muscle there is 5–8 mmol/l wet weight. Carnosine is one of the predominant buffers within the muscle. However, it may also have antioxidant properties and increase the calcium sensitivity of muscle, which is essential in producing a forceful contraction.

There are some natural indications of the importance of carnosine in preventing fatigue in high-intensity exercise. In other mammals, such as horses and greyhounds, which are bred for their ability to perform high-intensity exercise, skeletal muscle concentrations of carnosine are significantly higher than in humans. In humans, fast twitch muscle fibres tend to have a greater concentration of carnosine than slow twitch fibres. Likewise, humans who are trained for high-intensity exercise exhibit greater muscle carnosine concentrations than those who are endurance trained. As a side note, women tend to have a lower concentration of muscle carnosine than males, potentially due to a lower proportion of fast twitch fibres. We also tend to see a decrease in muscle carnosine concentration as we age.

Carnosine is made up of two amino acids, L-hisitidine and β-alanine. Carnosine content of the muscle is influenced by diet. Vegetarians have significantly lower muscle carnosine content than carnivores. This does make sense as carnosine is found predominantly in muscle, and of course vegetarians will not consume muscle in the form of meat. When

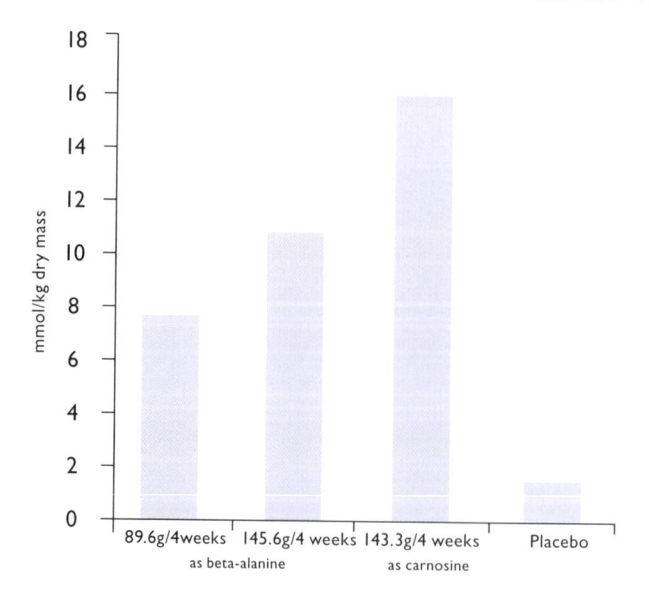

Increase in muscle carnosine content over four weeks of supplementation with different loading regimens compared to placebo (adapted from Harris et al., 2006).

EVENTS LASTING LESS THAN ONE HOUR AND WITH MULTIPLE ROUNDS

Change in total work done at 110 per cent maximum power output with placebo and β-alanine supplementation at four weeks and ten weeks of supplementation.

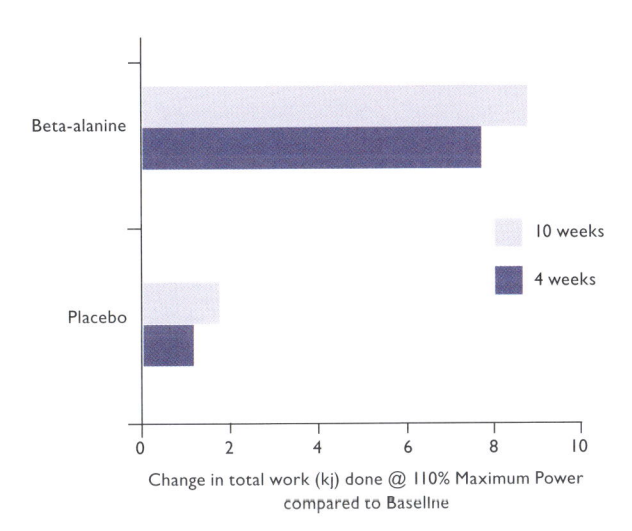

carnosine is consumed either through meat or supplementation, it is easily absorbed and is then broken down into its component amino acids, histidine and β-alanine.

It is thought that β-alanine is the rate-limiting step to synthesis of carnosine within the muscle. However, β-alanine alone does not occur in high amounts within a normal diet. Therefore, if there is a need to increase muscle carnosine, β-alanine needs to be supplemented.

Research led by a group headed by Roger Harris at Chichester University did just this. In an elegant series of studies the research group first showed that ingestion of β-alanine can increase muscle carnosine content of muscle. Ingestion of 4.8–6.0g of β-alanine daily increases muscle carnosine content by 60 per cent in four weeks, and 80 per cent in ten weeks of supplementation. Unlike creatine, the starting concentration of β-alanine makes no difference to how much of an increase can be seen.

So β-alanine supplementation increases muscle carnosine concentration in nearly everyone, and quite dramatically too. But does this increase exercise performance? Roger Harris's group set out to answer this question, too. Before and after ten weeks of β-alanine supplementation athletes performed a time to exhaustion trial at 110 per cent of VO_2 max. This is incredibly hard and causes fatigue in a matter of minutes. β-alanine supplementation improved time to fatigue by 8.6 per cent; in fact by four weeks of supplementation performance had been improved by 7.3 per cent. Interestingly, further analysis of the data from these studies showed the greater the increase in muscle carnosine content, the greater the increase in time to exhaustion.

Since these early research efforts to investigate the effect of β-alanine supplementation on exercise performance, there has been a whole series of studies continuing the research theme. Not all show an effect on performance, but a recent meta-analysis from the research group of Craig Sale at Nottingham Trent University shows a significant effect on performance of events that last between one and four minutes in duration. It is highly likely that in events lasting longer than four minutes, performance will be increased too according to the meta-analysis, but if the event is less than one minute in duration there is likely to be little effect.

In terms of dosing, it appears that there needs to be a total amount of approximately 180g of β-alanine ingested to increase muscle carnosine content and subsequently performance. However, taking this in one go would be difficult and potentially dangerous. One side effect of supplementing with β-alanine is a parathesia in the extremities – or in English, a strong tingling sensation in the face, fingers and toes. A dose under 10g and more practically 5g per day needs to be taken to reduce this side effect. Therefore a dose of around 3–5g per day for four weeks should be taken. Once muscle carnosine content is increased a maintenance dose of 1.5g per day is sufficient to maintain elevated concentrations. Once supplementation is ceased, the washout time is ten to twenty weeks, with positive performance effects remaining for up to six weeks.

Supplementing with β-alanine, therefore, increases muscle carnosine concentration to buffer more of the acid produced within the muscle itself. However, another technique can help to suck the hydrogen ions from the muscle into the blood, from where it can be disposed of. This technique involves simple baking soda, or sodium bicarbonate to give it its appropriate name.

Use of sodium bicarbonate to enhance exercise performance was first reported in the scientific literature by the legendary Fatigue Laboratory at Harvard University from the work of D.B. Dill's research group in 1931. As in many scientific experiments of this era, the researchers used themselves as guinea pigs. They first ingested ammonium chloride, thereby creating an acidic environment in their own bodies. Performance was decreased. In a second condition they supplemented with 10g of sodium bicarbonate. Here, performance was improved, giving the first indication that sodium bicarbonate could improve performance (although anyone familiar with using baking soda in baking will realize that 10g is far more than is normally used).

Bicarbonate naturally occurs within the blood, and is the major buffering component within the circulation. When you consume large amounts of sodium bicarbonate there is an increase in blood bicarbonate concentration. This causes an increase in the gradient for hydrogen ion transport between the muscle and the blood. This is easily seen in practice as, for a given exercise intensity, blood lactate will be higher when sodium bicarbonate has been supplemented – essentially making it easier for hydrogen ions to exit the muscle, a bit like increasing the speed of a river.

Once the hydrogen ion has entered the circulation it bonds with bicarbonate to form carbonic acid. From here carbonic acid is broken down into water and carbon dioxide. The carbon dioxide is exhaled through the lungs. Therefore, another potential marker of sodium bicarbonate supplementation is an increase in carbon dioxide of expired air.

The most common protocol to increase blood bicarbonate is to supplement with 0.3g/kg of body weight of sodium bicarbonate one to two hours prior to the start of the event. However, there are some potentially interesting side effects to using sodium bicarbonate. It is relatively common when ingesting large amounts of sodium bicarbonate in this way to induce a feeling of bloating in the stomach, stomach cramps and diarrhoea.

To reduce the side effects there are a number of approaches that could be tried. Firstly, the supplement should be consumed following a carbohydrate-based meal. As this is likely to be the pre-event meal, it should be easy to achieve. Secondly, smaller doses of 0.1–0.2g/kg of body weight could be supplemented over a longer period of time. Thirdly, sodium citrate could be used in a similar

EVENTS LASTING LESS THAN ONE HOUR AND WITH MULTIPLE ROUNDS

dosing protocol as it produces fewer side effects, although it is potentially a less potent buffer than sodium bicarbonate.

So after all this, what is the evidence that there is an effect on performance? There are as many studies which show a benefit as show no effect at all. A meta-analysis published in 2012 showed that on average, across forty studies that met the set criteria of inclusion, there was a small but significant effect on performance. It seems that there is more likely to be an effect on performance if the event lasts between one and ten minutes in duration; below or above this duration the effect decreases.

Recovery between rounds

Once a bout of exercise has been completed, what you eat, when you eat it and how much you eat affects the speed at which you recover from exercise. The first aspect to look at is the refilling of your fuel tank. In the case of exercising muscle, this is muscle glycogen.

When muscle glycogen is depleted post-exercise there is a potent push for the body to resynthesize muscle glycogen. Resynthesis of muscle glycogen occurs in preference to other glycogen stores such as in the liver. In the absence of carbohydrate intake and in order to provide the substrate for glycogen resynthesis, muscle will start the process of glycogen resynthesis through gluconeogenesis.

Let's look first of all at how the body promotes muscle glycogen resynthesis. In order to start the process of muscle glycogen resynthesis, glucose must be transported into the muscle cell. Glucose enters the muscle cell through the glucose transporter carrier proteins (GLUTs), of which there are many types. Two types are primarily found in muscle:

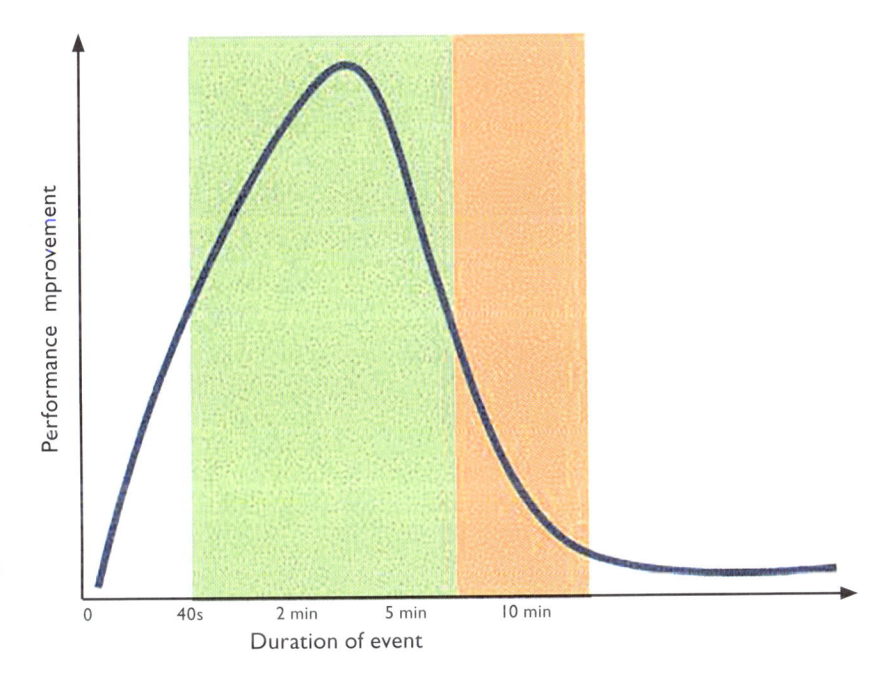

Schematic showing duration of event and conceptual effect on performance using nutritional buffers.

GLUT1 and GLUT4. However, GLUT4 is the one we need to focus on.

GLUT4 resides in vesicles that sit just below the cell's surface. Vesicles are small, fluid-based sacs that provide specific functions within a cell. When the muscle contracts the vesicles allow the movement of GLUT4 to the cell wall, where they can facilitate the transport of glucose into the muscle. However, once contractions are complete, GLUT4 slowly return to their vesicles, to the point where two hours later amounts of GLUT4 within the cell wall of a muscle can be returned to resting levels.

Exercise is not the only stimulus for the movement of GLUT4 from their vesicles to the cell wall. A second potent stimulator of this is the hormone insulin. When carbohydrates are consumed insulin is released in response in order to regulate blood glucose concentration. An increase in insulin will also promote the movement of GLUT4 from the vesicles within which they are held to the cell wall.

Upon entering the muscle cell, glucose is immediately converted to glucose-6-phosphate by the enzyme hexokinase. From here the process of glycogenesis occurs, with the primary limiting step being the activity of the enzyme glycogen synthase. When muscle glycogen concentrations are low, the activity of this enzyme is increased.

Phases of muscle glycogen resynthesis

So as we can see, glycogen resynthesis is regulated by the degree to which muscle glycogen is depleted, exercise and insulin. Post-exercise muscle glycogen repletion is characterized by two phases. The first is seen as the fast phase of muscle glycogen resynthesis and is independent of insulin. The primary reason for this is the increased GLUT4 concentration within the cell wall, as we have already seen. However, this first phase seems only to occur when muscle glycogen stores are below their threshold amount (seemingly around 128–150 mmol/kg of dry weight of muscle). This first phase has given rise to the term 'window of opportunity' or similar effective marketing slogans to ensure athletes consume carbohydrate in the post-exercise period.

The second phase of muscle glycogen resynthesis occurs at a slower rate, as high as a 50 per cent reduction in glycogen resynthesis post-exercise, but still higher than it would be pre-exercise. During this period of time, which in certain conditions can last up to forty-eight hours post-exercise, the muscle is more sensitive to the effects of the hormone insulin. It is more sensitive to the effects of insulin on the movement of GLUT4 to the cell wall, and to the effects of insulin increasing glycogen synthase activity.

Timing, type and amount of carbohydrate intake

We can start to see from the two-phase process of glycogen resynthesis that there will be a number of factors starting to influence how quickly muscle glycogen can be resynthesized. The first is timing of carbohydrate intake. By delaying intake of carbohydrate by just two hours after exercise, the rate at which muscle glycogen will be resynthesized will be slowed by 50 per cent. This delay in feeding will also reduce the available time to restore muscle glycogen before the next performance is needed.

Two excellent reviews over the last fifteen years on the topic of muscle glycogen resynthesis have come to a similar conclusion about the amount of carbohydrate to ingest to maximally resynthesize muscle glycogen. The first by Roy Jentjens in 2001, then a post-doctoral researcher at the University of Birmingham, seemed to show that 1g/kg of body weight per hour was optimal. This was backed up ten years later by James Betts from the

University of Bath, who with the addition to the analysis of the studies completed in that ten-year period was still able to show that this intake rate was optimal. It also seems that spreading this out into multiple smaller intakes of carbohydrate may be optimal throughout the initial hour post-exercise.

Within this initial period of muscle glycogen resynthesis, it appears that sugary, more simple carbohydrates will provide a greater rate of muscle glycogen resynthesis than more complex carbohydrates do. A study in the early 1990s from the Australian Institute of Sport showed that foods with a higher glycaemic index increase the rate of muscle glycogen resynthesis by approximately 30 per cent when compared to foods of a lower glycaemic index.

So far, we have seen that in order to maximally replenish muscle glycogen as quickly as possible we need to consume around 1g/kg of body weight of carbohydrate, starting as soon as possible post-exercise but splitting up this dose into smaller amounts and spreading the intake over the time period post-exercise.

One point to ensure is that muscle glycogen resynthesis is regulated by the degree to which muscle glycogen is depleted in the first instance. In some cases, such as during shorter events, muscle glycogen is unlikely to become depleted so an aggressive approach to muscle glycogen repletion is not necessary. Also, if there are more than eight hours between performances, and sufficient carbohydrate is consumed in the diet, muscle glycogen will be restored.

Addition of protein

Of course, generally single nutrients are not consumed independently. Along with carbohydrate there is a potential for the addition of protein to carbohydrate to improve muscle glycogen resynthesis too. While it seems that if high amounts of carbohydrate are consumed, the addition of protein to the mix will have very little effect on subsequent muscle glycogen repletion, at lower amounts, even at the rate of 1g per kg of body weight per hour, there appears to be some benefit to the addition of protein to the post-exercise recovery meal.

Why might this be? As we have seen, insulin has a potent effect on rates of muscle glycogen resynthesis. Carbohydrate is not the only nutrient that stimulates an insulin response. Protein does too, at times quite potently, seemingly in response to the appearance of certain amino acids in the circulation, in particular leucine, tyrosine and phenylalanine.

When protein is combined with carbohydrate in the post-exercise period, it appears that an amount of around 0.3g/kg of body weight is needed to augment this insulin response to the added protein. This follows the trend we saw in Chapter 3 for the amount needed to also maximally stimulate muscle protein synthesis.

So if the addition of protein to carbohydrate may in certain situations augment muscle glycogen resynthesis, what is the effect on subsequent exercise performance? There are actually very few studies that investigate the performance effect of maximizing the rate of muscle glycogen resynthesis post-exercise, and those studies that have done so have a number of limitations to their research design, including not matching the energy content of the drinks in the post-exercise period and using invalid protocols to assess performance after the recovery period.

In those studies that have investigated the effect of consuming carbohydrate with or without protein in the post-exercise period, it is clear that consuming these nutrients is superior to consuming nothing post-exercise. However, whether both need to be in tandem is debatable.

EVENTS LASTING LESS THAN ONE HOUR AND WITH MULTIPLE ROUNDS

Muscle soreness

Recovery from exercise may not be all about restoration of muscle glycogen, particularly in high-intensity exercise. Anyone who has completed high-intensity exercise is likely to have suffered the effects of post-exercise muscle soreness. This is a process where in the days after exercise muscles become painful at rest, but particularly when they contract. Walking can become painful and the thought of attacking stairs the stuff of nightmares. The pain generally increases over the first twenty-four hours after exercise, remains for up to seventy-two hours, and then starts to disappear. Along with muscle soreness comes a reduction in muscle function, which persists over a similar timeframe. This is usually assessed in the literature through the testing of a maximal voluntary contraction of the desired muscle groups.

What happens to cause this damage? Normally it is caused by eccentric-type exercise, where the muscle must lengthen and resist force at the same time. Changes begin to occur within the muscle fibre, and now we can start to see what has happened. A muscle fibre is made up a series of myofibrils, where the contractile mechanism of the muscle resides. These myofibrils appear to have a striated pattern of light and dark sections. The dark sections, or A band, are where two different types of fibres connect. Simply called thin and thick fibres, within the A band these fibres overlap and are connected by cross bridges, where the protein myosin on the thick filament connects with the protein actin on the thin filament. The light sections are where adjacent thick filaments connect along the myofibril. The point where adjacent fibres connect is termed the Z-line. It is here, at the Z-line, that damage due to exercise is particularly visible and remains so for up to seventy-two hours after exercise.

Muscle damage can be characterized by a flood of metabolites of muscle entering the circulation. Creatine kinase (CK) in particular has been picked on as a marker that can be used to monitor muscle damage, with significant increases in CK seen after damaging exercise. However, there is much debate about the validity of CK as a marker of muscle damage, as there are many factors that influence increases in CK within the circulation.

A further potential mechanism that causes soreness is the build-up of calcium within the muscle, which can be seen in response to damaging exercise. This activates a number of enzymes, which may start to break down proteins within the muscle and trigger an inflammatory cascade and subsequent pain.

Nutrients to reduce muscle soreness

The exact mechanisms by which certain exercise bouts cause pain and damage to muscle are unclear. However, can nutrition help to speed up this repair? Protein has been an obvious target of research. A whole range of approaches has been taken, from providing individual amino acids to ingesting mixtures of amino acids and whole proteins, such as whey proteins, to alleviate muscle soreness and enhance exercise recovery.

The research can be summarized quite easily. Generally, whether it's single amino acids or whole proteins, muscle soreness is reduced when protein is supplemented post-exercise. However, it is unclear whether some sort of protein supplementation enhances recovery of muscle function, as many studies were not able to observe significant differences. When the research is examined further, though, there does seem to be a general trend towards protein enhancing recovery post-exercise (with the numbers of participants within each study being potentially too low).

What might cause the reduction in soreness and the potential improvement in muscle recovery post-exercise? One theory is that it could be due to the increase in muscle protein synthesis, which is seen when protein is ingested. However, this is unlikely given the timeframe of recovery and the long time it takes to build new proteins.

A much more likely explanation may come from the influence of whey protein on satellite cell proliferation within muscle. Whenever muscle injury occurs, whether contraction induced in the case of muscle soreness or through some sort of trauma, satellite cells are essential in the repair of the damaged tissue. The more that are present, the more quickly the muscle will regenerate.

A research group from the University of Aarhus set out to study the effects of whey protein supplementation after damaging exercise on satellite cells in the recovery period. The group took twenty-four healthy

---

RESEARCH FOCUS

Cherry Juice and recovery

In 2006 a research team from the University of Vermont investigated the effects of cherry juice on muscle damage after damaging resistance exercise. For eight days prior to the exercise the participants consumed 354ml of Montmorency tart cherry juice or placebo. Over the next four days recovery in muscle strength was tracked.

The efficacy of supplementing with tart cherry juice was visible from twenty-four hours after the exercise bout had finished. Measuring muscle strength over these four days, when placebo was consumed there was a decrease in strength by 30 per cent, and after four days there was still a reduction of strength from baseline of 15 per cent. Whereas when cherry juice had been supplemented the decrease in strength twenty-four hours after exercise was only 10 per cent, and was back at baseline levels after three days.

Montmorency tart cherries are a naturally occurring source of polyphenols. Polyphenols are chemicals found in nature or through artificial synthesis that have multiples of phenol units in their chemical structure. This makes them potent antioxidants. They may also have specific functions within the body and are often classed as functional foods. They have several potential health effects, although many of them are not proven.

Since that first study by Connelly and colleagues from the University of Vermont, other studies have shown similar results. Much of this research has been conducted by the research group of Glynn Howatson at Northumbria University. The first of these studies looked at two groups completing the London Marathon. One group was supplemented with cherry juice for five days before the marathon while another group had a placebo. While a different exercise stimulus to the one in the Connelly study, a marathon was just as damaging. Those runners who used cherry juice prior to the race recovered muscle function more quickly in the days post-marathon; post-exercise inflammation was reduced and antioxidant capacity was increased.

Further to this study the Northumbria group looked at the effects of cherry juice and repeated days' cycling. For seven days trained cyclists consumed either a placebo or a cherry juice concentrate. On the last three days of supplementation the participants undertook 109 minutes of road cycling. Over a range of markers, cherry juice supplementation decreased those of oxidative stress and inflammation. This provides a possible mechanism to enhance recovery post-exercise.

volunteers and got them to perform a novel eccentric exercise task. Post-exercise, half of them consumed carbohydrate only, and the other consumed a mixture of whey protein and carbohydrate where the total calories were matched. The group that consumed the whey protein saw a doubling of the satellite cells present within their muscle fibres over the next seven days. Those that consumed carbohydrate saw no increase. These results give an indication of a plausible mechanism by which protein supplementation post-exercise may reduce soreness and increase muscle regeneration after damaging exercise.

As mentioned earlier, there may be an inflammatory effect that causes muscle soreness post-exercise as well as a mechanical one. As such, nutrients that have an anti-inflammatory effect have been researched to look at their effects on post-exercise muscle soreness. The effects of these were subject to a Cochrane Review by Dr Mayur Ranchordas of Sheffield Hallam University in 2012. A whole range of interventions was used to study the effects of anti-inflammatory nutrients on exercise recovery. The review showed that for those who took the approach of supplementing with high doses of single vitamins, like vitamins C and E, there seemed to be no effect. Foods such as Montmorency cherries or pomegranates, however, seemed to have an effect. While the reason for this is not clear at present, it is likely to be due to the high polyphenol content of these types of food, which have potent anti-inflammatory effects within the body.

Summary

- Increased appearance of lactate in the blood often characterizes high-intensity exercise.
- Increases in lactate production can be seen as a marker of an increase in acid production due to high rates of energy production through glycolysis.
- Lactate per se is not inhibiting of muscle contraction. It is merely a store of carbohydrates by the body to be used at a later time.
- Increases in pH in the muscle can cause fatigue. Nutritional interventions can influence how the body buffers the acid produced through glycolysis.

Gold

Beta-alanine: Supplementation with 4–6g per day of beta-alanine increases the presence of the muscle buffer carnosine. Performance will be improved in events lasting between one and four minutes and likely in events up to ten minutes.

Sodium bicarbonate: Supplementing with 0.3g per kg of body weight ninety minutes prior to the start of an event lasting between one and ten minutes in duration will lead to an improvement in performance.

Carbohydrate post-exercise: Consuming 1g of quickly absorbed carbohydrates per kg of body weight immediately after exercise, broken into two or three feeds, will maximize muscle glycogen resynthesis.

Silver

Protein intake post-exercise: 0.3g of protein per kg of body weight taken post-exercise may promote muscle repair and regeneration and therefore promote recovery.

Cherry juice: Contains high amounts of polyphenols. These may help the muscle to recover more quickly after damaging exercise.

EVENTS LASTING LESS THAN ONE HOUR AND WITH MULTIPLE ROUNDS

Table 8.1 Example diet plan for Chapter 8.

Meal	Food
Breakfast	Large bowl of porridge made with semi-skimmed milk, with walnuts and raspberries 125g pot of Greek yogurt 1 apple 1 probiotic yogurt Cup of tea with milk
Post-Exercise	20g of whey protein with 35g of carbohydrates 1 banana
Lunch	1 tin of tuna with a baked sweet potato and a mixed salad
Snack	2 slices of wholemeal bread with almond butter
Post-Exercise	1 pint of semi-skimmed milk made into a smoothie with blueberries
Dinner	1 chicken breast with brown rice, broccoli, kale and carrots
Pre-bed snack	125g pot of Greek yogurt with berries

Carbohydrate (g/kg body weight)	Protein (g/kg body weight)	Fat (g/kg body weight)
4.2	2.3	1.2

Further reading

Beelen, M., Burke, L., Gibala, M. J. & van Loon, L. J. C. (2010). Nutritional strategies to promote postexercise recovery. *International Journal of Sport Nutrition and Exercise Metabolism* 1–17.

Burke, L. M. (2008). Caffeine and sports performance. *Applied Physiology, Nutrition, and Metabolism = Physiologie Appliquée, Nutrition et Métabolisme*, 33(6), 1319–34. doi:10.1139/H08-130

Jentjens, R. & Jeukendrup, A. (2003). Determinants of post-exercise glycogen synthesis during short-term recovery. *Sports Medicine (Auckland, N.Z.)*, 33(2), 117–44.

McNaughton, L., Backx, K., Palmer, G. & Strange, N. (1999). Effects of chronic bicarbonate ingestion on the performance of high-intensity work. *European Journal of Applied Physiology and Occupational Physiology*, 80(4), 333–6.

Rollo, I., & Williams, C. (2011). Effect of Mouth-Rinsing Carbohydrate Solutions on Endurance Performance. *Sports Medicine*, 41(6), 449–461.

CHAPTER 9

IMPROVING TEAM SPORT PERFORMANCE

Deep into injury time, the ball is swung in from the right side of the pitch. The big centre-half gets up for the ball. He's not jumped quite high enough, and the ball floats over his head. The full-back wasn't expecting that. He mis-controls the ball, and it squirms away from him. The opponents' substitute striker reacts. In one fluid movement of his body he controls the ball with his left foot, moves it towards his right, where with a little back lift he hits the ball with such power it sends the net rippling, straining backwards. He peels away towards his team's fans, one hand in the air, and a look on his face that shows he knows he has just scored the winning goal in a Cup final. The defenders are on their knees. The big centre-half is lying on the turf, head in his hands, devastated that one little error in concentration has caused his team to lose.

In one way or another, in a team sport this is a relatively common occurrence. It is well established that in a sport like football, more goals are scored in the last ten minutes of a match than in any other ten-minute period of the whole ninety minutes. This is backed up by other stats, which show evidence of fatigue towards the end of a football match. The number of times a player gets the ball and then passes it on is reduced in the final ten minutes. More short passes generally occur in the first half than in the second in many leagues around the world.

Clearly, there is a strong indication that skill performance is reduced towards the end of a match. However, so is physical performance. There are fewer high-intensity movements as the match continues, and it is not just soccer where this type of challenge occurs. Match analyses reveal that rugby matches, both league and union, show evidence of reductions in physical and skill performance late in the second half, once again leading to the potential for mistakes to occur and matches to be lost.

Carbohydrates

Where physiological measurements have taken place in either simulated or actual match play, it is clear that there is a significant demand on muscle glycogen as a fuel source during football. Consistently the evidence shows that over the course of a ninety-minute match muscle glycogen concentration can be reduced by up to 50 per cent compared to the starting level, with the effect more pronounced in fast twitch muscle fibres. This is backed up by the more acidic environment found within the muscle after football matches, giving a strong indication that glycolysis has been the predominant

IMPROVING TEAM SPORT PERFORMANCE

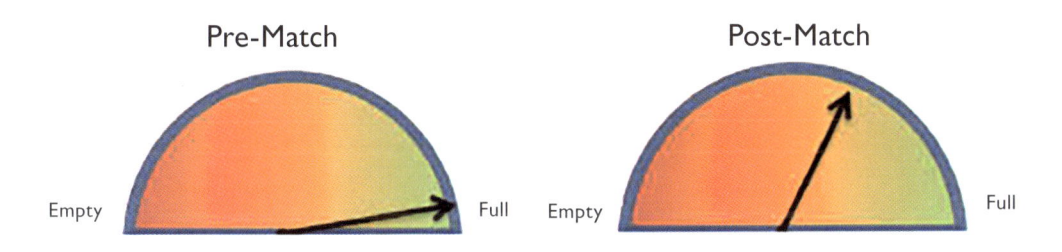

Pre-Match   **Post-Match**

Muscle glycogen status before and after a football match (adapted from Krustrup et al., 2006).

source of energy production. These factors combine to explain the reduction in sprint performance as a football match progresses.

From what we know, it seems the reduction in muscle glycogen presents a significant and valid route by which fatigue can occur. As we saw in Chapter 7, improving endurance performance by increasing carbohydrate intake prior to exercise performance can lead to an increase in muscle glycogen concentrations and subsequently performance.

Jens Bangsbo, one of the eminent researchers in the field of football performance and a former assistant manager at Juventus in Italy, was one of the first to look at carbohydrate loading in the context of team sports. His research group simulated the physical elements of football between field-based, intermittent running and a treadmill exercise test to exhaustion. On one occasion the participants consumed a diet that contained approximately 8g of carbohydrate per kg of body weight, while in the second condition they only consumed 4.5g per kg of body weight for two days prior to the test.

Those who consumed the higher-carbohydrate diet increased total running distance by 5 per cent compared to when the lower-carbohydrate diet was consumed. Other research has shown a similar pattern of increased distance covered with a higher carbohydrate intake in the days leading into a match.

From the research based around endurance exercise, an increase in muscle glycogen content can be achieved with only one day of increased carbohydrate intake. Therefore, the day before a match an intake of 8g of carbohydrate per kg of body weight will be sufficient to increase muscle glycogen content and therefore physical performance throughout the match.

While increasing carbohydrate content in the lead-up to a match can improve physical performance, carbohydrate ingested during a match seems to improve skill performance.

In 2004 I was fortunate enough to lead a research project looking at how carbohydrate intake immediately before and during a simulated football match improves skill performance throughout. I was a PhD student at the time and this was a way for me to learn about conducting research. Aided by an undergraduate student, Steve Conway, a talented footballer himself, we set out to find the answer.

Steve had the contacts to pull in the university football team for the trials. We set up a physical simulation of a football match: two halves of forty-five minutes, lots of change of pace and direction running, which we recorded onto an audio CD so we could keep the timings consistent. Before each half and twice within them we put the participants through four different tests: a test of agility, a test of dribbling skill, jump height and shooting accuracy.

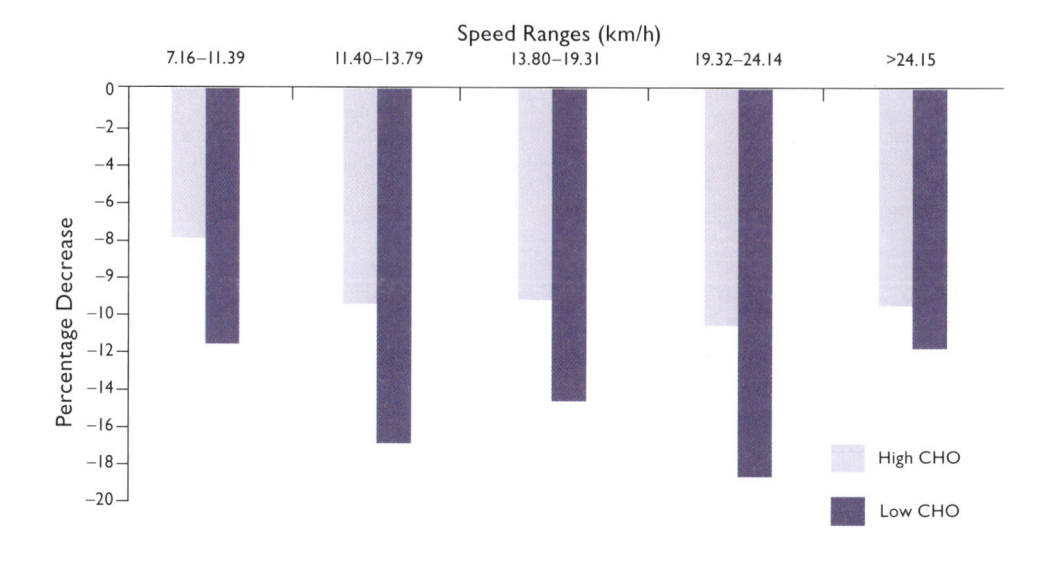

Percentage decrease in distance covered second half versus first half on a high- (High CHO) or low-carbohydrate (Low CHO) diet (adapted from Souglis et al., 2013).

On one occasion the participants consumed flavoured water. On a second occasion they consumed a sports drink throughout. Agility, dribbling performance and shooting accuracy were improved by 2.0 per cent, 3.2 per cent and 3.4 per cent respectively. No effect on jump height performance was seen. The improvement in performance in all cases occurred during the second half of the simulated match when fatigue was beginning to occur.

Other studies have shown a similar effect of ingesting carbohydrate during a simulated football match. These studies have also shown an attenuation in the reduction in shooting power seen during match play, and an improvement in passing accuracy with carbohydrate intake during a match. Similar effects have been shown in rugby-specific simulations, too.

However, simulated matches are fine but taking on board carbohydrate during a match is not always easy. Half-time intake of carbohydrates, therefore, needs to be maximized. As at half-time there is likely to be a need to take in large amounts of carbohydrate, it is worth considering using a carbohydrate drink that contains a mixture of multiple transportable carbohydrates to maximize absorption of those carbohydrates and minimize gastrointestinal distress. Players could also take on board carbohydrates if there are breaks in play on the field, such as for an injury. It is clear that carbohydrate intake during matches will increase physical and skill performances in team sports.

Recovery between matches

As we saw from the discussion around fatigue in football performance, there is significant

IMPROVING TEAM SPORT PERFORMANCE

glycogen depletion. Along with this glycogen depletion, other factors contribute to a decrease in physical performance in the days following a football match. Given that at professional levels there is often a need to complete two matches a week, with only two to three days in between, recovery between matches is essential to overall football performance.

Like recovery from any exercise bout, it can be considered in parts. The first, traditional view is to look at changes in the periphery, so in the muscles themselves. The second is to look at the brain and the role of the central nervous system. There is often a disconnect between the two as they recover at different speeds.

After a football match, if a player is forced to produce a maximal contraction and the force of that contraction is measured, there will be an immediate decrease in the force compared to prior to the match. Over the next twenty-four hours the force the player is able to apply increases, but will not reach baseline levels. However, if at baseline and twenty-four hours later the muscle was to be electrically stimulated to contract, the force would be similar. This suggests that force can be recovered at the point of the muscle, but a recovery of the brain and nervous system is much slower. Unfortunately, it is also not as clearly understood.

Carbohydrate and recovery

The research group of Jens Bangsbo in Copenhagen, Denmark, set out to investigate whether a diet that provided macronutrient proportions of 71 per cent carbohydrate, 21 per cent protein and 8 per cent fat would provide superior recovery in muscle glycogen concentrations following a football match. This was compared to a diet in the forty-eight hours post-match of 55 per cent carbohydrate, 18 per cent protein and 26 per cent fat.

There was no difference in muscle glycogen forty-eight hours later. However, this should not be too surprising as high amounts of carbohydrate are only really needed if there are less than twenty-four hours to replace muscle glycogen.

Football-type exercise does provide a challenge to high rates of muscle glycogen resynthesis in the post-exercise period. A significant amount of muscle damage occurs during a football match, and in other sports where the movements are intermittent in nature. Muscle damage seems to reduce the rate of muscle glycogen resynthesis in the immediate post-exercise period. A Swiss research group headed by Monica Zehnder showed that despite ingesting a very high-carbohydrate diet in the post-exercise period, muscle damage caused a further decrease in muscle glycogen compared to non-damaged exercise controls. Those who performed the damaging exercise took forty-eight hours to fully restore muscle glycogen, whereas those who performed non-damaging exercise took only twenty-four hours.

Milk and recovery

It is clear that damaging muscle causes a slowing of muscle glycogen resynthesis. Therefore, a priority in recovery from team sport exercise should be the repair of muscle damage. A series of studies looking at milk provides a fascinating insight into how food can do just this.

Emma Cockburn, a PhD student at Northumbria University, set out in her PhD studies to look at the role of milk intake in recovery from damaging exercise. In the first of the series, participants undertook exercise on an isokinetic dynamometer. If you don't know what these are, they look a bit like a machine out of *Rocky 4*. However, they are a good way of providing a controlled muscle contraction. They also allow for eccentric contractions to take place, and these are a surefire way to elicit muscle damage. After this exercise, the participants were provided with one litre of four different drinks: water, milk, a milk-based recovery shake that included more carbohydrate than milk alone, or a standard carbohydrate sports drink. So while the volume was the same, there were differences in nutritional make-up of the four drinks.

Perceptive markers of muscle soreness were assessed after the damage for the next two days. While statistical significance was not reached, there was a trend for the subjective markers of muscle soreness to be reduced when milk was ingested. The ability to produce force was also assessed, and both the milk drinks and the milk-based recovery drink prevented a drop-off in force for the forty-eight hours after the exercise. Those who drank the carbohydrate drink and only water produced less force twenty-four hours later, and even less force a further day later. Both the milk drink and milk-based recovery drink also attenuated a rise in creatine kinase for the two days after the exercise, whereas when only the carbohydrate drink or water were drunk the creatine kinase in the circulation increased by ten- and twenty-fold respectively two days later.

So milk seems to attenuate muscle damage, whether it be in the form of milk or a milk-based recovery shake containing added carbohydrate. The next study from Northumbria University assessed the effect of timing of the milk-based recovery drink. This time 1 litre of a milk recovery drink, containing 707 kcal, 33.4g of protein, 118.2g of carbohydrate and 16.4g of fat, was consumed before damaging exercise, immediately after exercise, twenty-four hours after the exercise or not at all.

Consuming the drink before or after the exercise certainly seemed to reduce muscle soreness compared to not consuming the milk at all. When looking at the ability to produce force in the ensuing days, something interesting seems to happen. Both at forty-eight hours and seventy-two hours after the exercise, consuming the milk immediately afterwards and twenty-four hours afterwards attenuated the loss of force seen, with taking the milk immediately after the exercise being superior to twenty-four hours later. However, consuming the milk before the exercise seemed to have minimal effect. As with many aspects of sports nutrition, timing seems to be key, and consuming the milk immediately after exercise as normal is the optimal time to do it to reduce muscle damage.

Drinking nearly two pints of milk is not easy, so the next study looked at the volume needed. The same damaging exercise was performed, and immediately after the exercise the participants drank either 500ml, 1,000ml, or 1,000ml of water. There appeared to be no differences between the drinks in terms of muscle soreness. However, both 500ml and 1,000ml of milk attenuated the loss of force produced by the muscle in the seventy-two hours after the exercise. It seems 500ml of milk is just as effective as 1,000ml of milk in reducing muscle damage and enhancing recovery.

In this initial series of studies, the measure of performance was in a laboratory-controlled situation. For the final study in the series, measures similar to those needed for team sport performance were used. Measures such as jump height, agility and sprint time were assessed along with performance of the Loughborough Intermittent Shuttle Test (LIST), a controlled assessment of team sport-type performance. After the damaging exercise, the participants consumed either 500ml of milk or water.

Three days after the damaging exercise was performed, consuming milk was speeding up recovery. Speed over 15m was 5.9 per cent slower three days later when only water was consumed, whereas speed had only reduced by 2.6 per cent when milk was drunk. Participants were more agile three days later, their scores on the agility test were back to baseline, whereas with water they were still reduced by 4.8 per cent. Using the LIST as a measure of repeated sprint performance, two days after the damaging exercise repeated sprint performance was back to baseline in those who consumed milk. In those who didn't, their repeated sprint performance was reduced by 2.4 per cent.

It seems highly likely that milk can enhance recovery after damaging exercise. It would be interesting in the future to see if it is milk itself that causes the improved recovery, or just the presence of carbohydrates and proteins within the milk.

Antioxidants and recovery

One interesting area to consider is the use of antioxidants. Alterations in redox balance can influence performance and recovery. Redox balance is influenced by oxidative stress and antioxidant status. Oxidative stress is driven by the production of reactive oxygen species (ROS). ROS are produced in response to exercise and can cause fatigue, and also have an influence in the adaptive response to exercise.

One promising supplement to influence redox balance is N-acetyl-cysteine (NAC). Once entered into the circulation, the acetyl group is removed and cysteine is released. Cysteine supports glutathione synthesis, which is essential in maintaining redox balance.

A recent study in 2011 from Liverpool John Moores University tested the effect of supplementing with 100mg of NAC per kg per day over a six-day period. On days two, four and six, the participants performed the LIST mentioned earlier along with the Yo-Yo Intermittent Recovery Test level 1 (YIRT-1); on days three and five tests of muscle function were performed.

Those who consumed the NAC appeared to recovery more effectively. The YIRT-1 performance reduced in those consuming placebo, but increased in those consuming NAC. Twenty-metre sprint times during the LIST were also more effectively maintained when NAC was supplemented compared to placebo.

These results show a promising role for NAC supplementation in enhancing recovery from team sport exercise. However, it should be noted that some individuals reported gastrointestinal distress in response to ingested NAC, so it is important that this intervention is trialled prior to use.

Sleep

Team sports often require multiple matches per week. Sleep will therefore become an important part of recovery.

Your head hits the pillow. Your eyes close. All snug and warm. It's time to get a good night's sleep. I will drop off anytime soon. Anytime, really. Oh no, why can't I get to sleep? We've all been through situations where it is difficult to drop off to sleep, whether it's because of jet lag, stress at work or some other, unknown reason.

Sleep is one of the most important processes the body goes through, and along with eating and exercise is one of the things humans do daily (well, we all should exercise anyway). On average, humans get seven or eight hours' sleep per night. Sleep is split into two primary phases, rapid eye movement (REM) and non-rapid eye movement (NREM), which has three stages. Sleep generally proceeds through the three stages of NREM and is followed by a stage of REM. This process is repeated four or five times per night.

How important is sleep to an athlete? It seems it is very important. In studies where participants have been restricted from sleeping for twenty-four hours or more, the effects on performance are clear. There is a reduction in pretty much all types of performance, whether it's reaction time, speed, strength or endurance.

However, the evidence for partial disturbance in sleep is not as strong. There does seem to be some suggestion that consistently getting poor sleep can affect endurance performance more than strength performance.

There are, however, other consequences of consistently poor sleep that will affect an athlete. Primarily the negative effects of sleep deprivation on cognitive function, an increase in sensitivity to pain, decreases in immune function and increased appetite could all lead to negative effects on performance.

So how does what you eat affect sleep? In some cases the evidence is unclear. It seems from a whole diet point of view that a high-carbohydrate diet will allow you to get to sleep quicker, a high-protein diet will keep you asleep for longer, and a high-fat diet will decrease sleep duration. In essence it seems there is little evidence for one type of diet being better than another to promote sleep, with all affecting it in different ways. One key factor, though, appears to be consuming sufficient energy. A calorie-deficit diet has a tendency to lead towards lower-quality sleep.

Acute interventions seem to be more successful. These focus around the biochemical pathways that promote sleep. One of the neurotransmitters that leads to sleep is serotonin. Serotonin is the precursor of the hormone melatonin, which can be thought of as the master switch of sleep.

Serotonin is produced from the amino acid tryptophan. Tryptophan is one of the least abundant amino acids consumed by the body. It also has competition to cross the blood–brain barrier, where it can be converted into serotonin and subsequently melatonin. It is in competition with tyrosine and the branched-chain amino acids in particular. The other amino acids are more abundant in the diet and therefore often win the battle to cross the blood–brain barrier.

One simple solution seems to be increasing the dietary content of tryptophan to promote sleep. Doses of tryptophan as low as 1g promote a decrease in sleep latency and an increase in sleep quality. Essentially, you will get to sleep more quickly, and spend more time having good-quality sleep.

High-glycaemic acid carbohydrates can also help you get off to sleep more quickly. Rapidly absorbed carbohydrates, with sugar being the simplest form, promote a spike in the hormone insulin. This increase in insulin stores the amino acids that compete with tryptophan in muscle. This therefore increases tryptophan in relation to its competing amino acids and more is available to cross the blood–brain barrier and produce serotonin. Carbohydrate ingestion up to an hour prior to sleep does seem to decrease the time it takes to get to sleep. However, be warned – if you consume this too close to sleep, within one hour, then you are more likely to stay awake for longer.

Travel

Athletes often have to travel around the world to compete. This can be a challenge to their ability to consume the appropriate foods. Athletes should start preparing for travel well ahead of departure, assuming the travel will involve flying to a different destination, taking time to plan what food they might need to take with them on their journey.

IMPROVING TEAM SPORT PERFORMANCE

While on the plane, food may not be optimal but where possible athletes should try to get into the rhythm of food intake similar to their destination. Care should be taken to monitor hydration; there may be a need to either purchase or take on board fluid on top of what's available in-flight.

With air travel there is often a change in time zones, with the potential for jet lag. This can have a knock-on effect on food intake, in particular appetite and metabolic and physiologic responses to food. The body's circadian rhythm or body clock is driven by cells located at the base of the hypothalamus in the brain. The natural day/night cycle provides the largest stimulus to drive the body clock, with the hormone melatonin in particular being released as light turns into dark.

There are many consequences to the body's natural rhythms, with changes in metabolism and even sports performance evident depending on the time of day. Food provides another signal for the body to maintain its natural rhythms and there are some changes that affect our responses to food depending on the time of day. For instance, there is a reduction in blood flow to the gut and intestine in the evening once it becomes dark, which may lead to a slowing of digestion following food intake. This may induce a feeling of being bloated, which could affect sleep.

There have been a number of potential 'diets' proposed that may help with jet lag, although many of these have little direct evidence behind them. One of the well-known ones is the Argonne diet, where for four days prior to departure you alternate days between fasting and feasting.

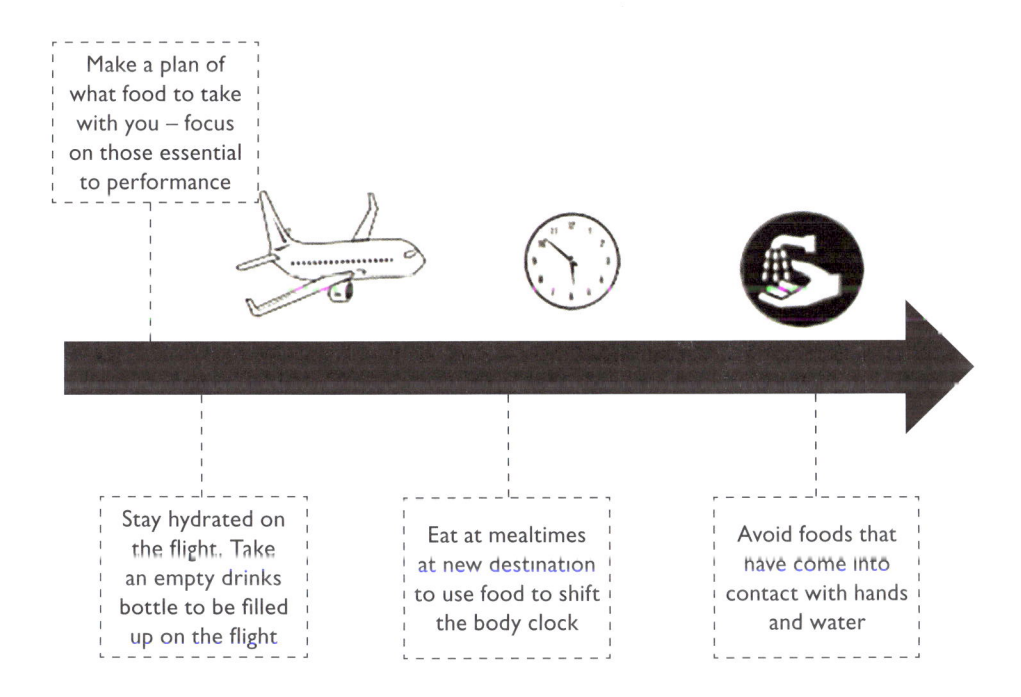

Key nutrition aspects of travel for an athlete.

IMPROVING TEAM SPORT PERFORMANCE

On arrival, and particularly if a number of time zones have been crossed, the biggest stimulation for adapting to the new time zone is exposure to light. However, there is also some potential for food to provide a small effect. There are some theories around manipulating the availability of the amino acids tyrosine and tryptophan, depending on the time of day. Tyrosine stimulates arousal, while tryptophan stimulates drowsiness.

In theory, tyrosine concentrations in the blood will increase after ingestion of protein-based meals, with tryptophan concentrations increasing after ingestion of carbohydrate-based meals. Therefore, there have been some suggestions that breakfast meals should be based around protein and evening meals around carbohydrate to manipulate tyrosine and tryptophan concentrations. However, there is minimal evidence to support this, and an athlete's meal timings and concentrations should be driven by their training and competition schedule on arrival at a new destination.

A further factor to consider while travelling is food hygiene. It is not uncommon for athletes to contract a gastrointestinal infection; travellers' diarrhoea is common. This may be the case when travelling to countries where food hygiene standards are not as good as those in Western countries. The main areas of concern are with foods that have come into contact with water, or that could have come into contact with a person's hands, or food not being served at a hot enough temperature.

Summary

- Team sports are won and lost by effective use of skill and decision-making under fatigue and pressure. Nutrition can help this process.
- Fatigue occurs towards the end of team sport competitions, with a reduction in passing accuracy and a reduction in high-intensity movements in the last ten minutes of football matches.
- Muscle glycogen provides a key source of energy during football matches, with reductions of up to 50 per cent of starting muscle glycogen concentration in some football matches.
- Sleep is an important part of recovery. A number of nutrients may influence how an athlete sleeps.
- Travel is an important part of performing at the elite level. Crossing time zones and competing in different environments can be a challenge for athletes.

Gold
Carbohydrate loading: Consume 8g of carbohydrate per kg of body weight for the day before a match to increase muscle glycogen concentrations.

Carbohydrate intake during: Where match play and stoppages allow, consuming between 30 and 60g of carbohydrates per half will delay fatigue during football-type matches. This will also allow better skill performance.

Caffeine: Although discussed primarily in Chapter 6 on nutrition and brain function, it appears that 1–3mg of caffeine prior to a match will lead to greater skill performance.

Silver
Carbohydrate post-exercise: Consuming 1g per kg of body weight immediately post-match will lead to optimal rates of muscle glycogen resynthesis. This will enhance recovery, and therefore allow the player to train or play as soon as possible.

Milk: Consuming 500ml of milk immediately

IMPROVING TEAM SPORT PERFORMANCE

Table 9.1 Example diet plan for Chapter 9.

Meal	Food
Breakfast	Large bowl of porridge made with semi-skimmed milk, with walnuts and raspberries 125g pot of Greek yogurt 1 apple 1 probiotic yogurt Cup of tea with milk 1 bagel with jam
During Exercise	2–3 isotonic carbohydrate gel and 750ml of 6% carbohydrate electrolyte drink
Post-Exercise	20g of whey protein with 35g of carbohydrates made with 500ml of milk 1 apple
Lunch	1 tin of tuna with a baked sweet potato and a mixed salad
Snack	2 slices of wholemeal bread with almond butter
Post-Exercise	1 pint of semi-skimmed milk made into a smoothie with blueberries
Dinner	1 chicken breast with brown rice, broccoli, kale and carrots
Pre-bed snack	1 125g pot of Greek yogurt with berries

Carbohydrate (g/kg body weight) 6.3	Protein (g/kg body weight) 2.3	Fat (g/kg body weight) 0.9

after a match will enhance recovery post-match. Milk may be particularly useful in promoting recovery from damaging exercise.

High-GI foods pre-bed: Consuming sugary foods prior to going to bed may promote sleep.

Tryptophan: Doses as low as 1g of tryptophan may promote sleep. Some foods are naturally high in tryptophan.

Bronze
NAC: Antioxidants such as NAC provided in a dose of 100mg per kg of body weight per day for six days may improve muscle recovery from damaging exercise.

Further reading

Cobley, J. N., McGlory, C., Morton, J. P. & Close, G. L. (2011). N-Acetylcysteine's attenuation of fatigue after repeated bouts of intermittent exercise: practical implications for tournament situations. *International Journal of Sport Nutrition and Exercise Metabolism*, 21(6), 451–61.

Cockburn, E., Bell, P. G. & Stevenson, E. (2013). Effect of Milk on Team Sport Performance following Exercise-Induced Muscle Damage. *Medicine and Science in Sports and Exercise.* doi:10.1249/MSS.0b013e31828b7dd0

Currell, K., Conway, S. & Jeukendrup, A. E. (2009). Carbohydrate ingestion improves performance of a new reliable test of soccer performance. *International Journal of Sport Nutrition and Exercise Metabolism,* 19(1), 34–46.

Russell, M. & Kingsley, M. (2014). The efficacy of acute nutritional interventions on soccer skill performance. *Sports Medicine* (Auckland, N.Z.), 44(7), 957–70.

Souglis, A. et al. (2013). The effect of high-vs. low-carbohydrate diets on distances covered in soccer. *Journal of Strength and Conditioning Research.* 27(8). 2235-2247.

CHAPTER 10

WEIGHT MANAGEMENT

'Oh no, my weight has gone up again. I can't believe it! Every day I step on the scales it changes. I weigh myself in the morning, then in the afternoon, and it's gone up. Then the next day it goes up again. I am trying so hard to lose weight, yet whatever I do nothing changes.'

I would say the above quote is typical of many athletes, or even non-athletes. Weight loss is the most common reason an athlete might engage with a nutritionist, although I hope that you have seen throughout this book that nutrition impacts on so much more than just weight loss. However, there are often legitimate reasons why an athlete might want to lose some weight.

What is body weight composed of?

Let's start at the beginning. What makes up body weight? Firstly, let's break it down into some of the functional components of the human body for a typical 70kg male human. Approximately 42 per cent is muscle, so 29.4kg of muscle. This is higher for athletes; strength and power athletes often have greater than 50 per cent muscle mass. About 12–15 per cent of the average male will be made up of body fat, so about 9kg in total. The skeleton weighs somewhere in the region of 16 per cent of male weight, so 11kg for our average man. The brain weighs approximately 1.5kg, as does the liver, the lungs 0.4kg each, along with a heart's weight of approx. 0.3kg. The other organs all weigh between 0.1 and 0.2kg. Blood accounts for approximately 5kg of weight, but could be more in endurance athletes due to the increase in blood volume seen with endurance training. Of course we have not even included the stomach, intestines or their contents, or even the contents of the bladder.

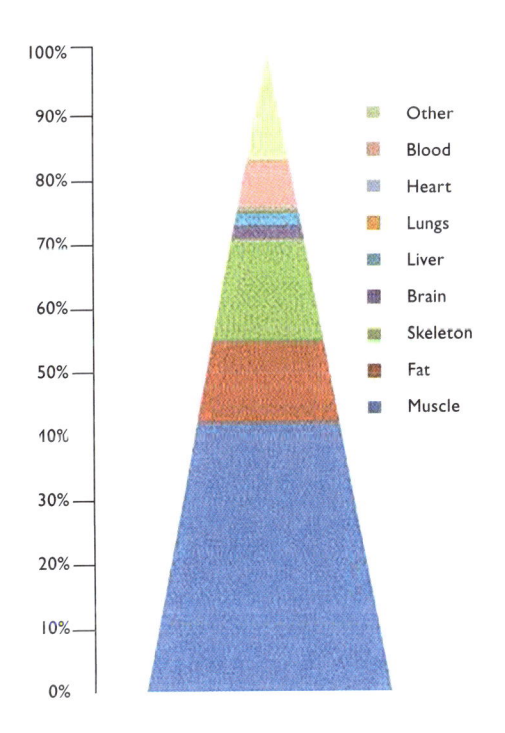

Percentage of body weight for different components of the body.

129

WEIGHT MANAGEMENT

As is clear from the above, body weight is made up of a large variety of components, all of which can contribute to changes in weight. Changes in a handful of these can account for variation in body weight, especially in those who exercise regularly. Water makes up the largest component of the human body, approximately 50–70 per cent. It is not uncommon during exercise for this water component to decrease by over 5 per cent due to sweat loss. Similarly, the glycogen content of muscles and the liver fluctuates depending on exercise. Moreover every 1 gram of glycogen is stored with 3 grams of water. So for example, if during exercise an athlete used 200g of muscle glycogen + 50g of liver glycogen this would mean they would lose 1kg of weight. On the flipside to this an adaptation to endurance training is an increase in muscle glycogen concentration by up to 50 per cent, so this could be a theoretical increase in body weight due to an increase in muscle glycogen concentration of 800g. Endurance training also increases blood volume by anything up to 0.5kg. It is clear, therefore, that body weight is variable.

Shape, size and performance

To understand the effects of an athlete's shape and size on performance we need to look at athletics performance in the same way Charles Darwin looked upon the natural world. We must look at what is already happening around us. As running is the most natural of all exercise, this is a good place to start.

Marathon and 10,000m runners tend to be the shortest, with an increase in height seen as the distance decreases until 400m, from where there is a slight decrease in height to those running 200m and 100m. Therefore 400m runners tend to be the tallest, and endurance runners the shortest.

Why would this be so? With an increase in height is likely to come an increase in stride length, and as running speed is simply stride length multiplied by stride frequency it is easy to see that an increase in stride length will lead to an increase in speed. Indeed, it is hypothesized that an increase of centre of gravity by 3 per cent leads to an increase in running speed of 1.5 per cent.

Sprinters tend to be shorter than 400m runners. This is likely to be a function of too much height decreasing stride frequency. So while stride length is increased, stride frequency is decreased and therefore there is no increase in speed. However, the success of recent sprinters such as Usain Bolt (1.95m tall) may be due to an ability to maintain an adequate stride frequency with the already natural advantage of a long stride length. There is also a possibility that a shorter athlete may be better able to react to the starting gun and have a lower moment of inertia to be able to accelerate to top speed.

However, athletes cannot alter their height in the same way that they can alter their body mass. From theories of animal locomotion it seems evident that speed increases with the mass of the animal. A similar trend is clear in human movement too: body mass tends to be greatest in 100m runners, and decreases as a function of distance up until marathon running.

Greater mass in sprinters is likely to have a performance effect by increasing efficiency of sprinting through an increase in muscle strength, ground reaction forces and power. There is also likely to be a greater return of elastic energy through the stretch-shortening cycle. Indeed, looking at weights of Olympic champion sprinters compared to mere finalists, the champions tend to be heavier.

WEIGHT MANAGEMENT

For endurance runners the inverse seems true. A decrease in body mass will lead to an increase in endurance performance. From a mechanical perspective this will be a function of an increase in economy of movement, a major determinant of endurance performance (see Chapter 5) and an increase in mechanical efficiency. Interestingly, there will also be a decrease in ground reaction forces. This decrease in ground reaction forces will be important for runners undertaking high volumes of training as it may well be protective against injury and allow them to complete these high training volumes.

For endurance runners other benefits may come from a reduction in body mass:

- A reduction in overall body size through mass reduction will lead to a decrease in air resistance at a given speed. As many elite marathon runners are running at a pace well over 20km/h this will be significant.
- Gravity is the greatest force that needs to overcome with running, and of course a reduction in body mass will reduce the force needed to overcome gravity.
- Heavier runners will probably reach their heat storage limit sooner than those who are lighter. A decrease in body mass does confer a thermoregulatory advantage. This is important in hot environments as well as more temperate where the duration of metabolic energy turnover will produce heat that needs to be dissipated.

Body Mass Index (BMI) also provides an interesting insight into the link between shape size and performance. Nature normally encourages diversity. However, BMI shows an interesting trend for a decrease in diversity within a given running distance.

BMI increases as a function of running speed between distances. Male sprinters tend to have the highest BMI, with an average in world-leading athletes of 24.5kg/m^2, leading up to an elite male marathon runner having an average BMI of 19.5kg/m^2. However, within each discipline the variation between individuals' BMI decreases as a function of standard. For instance, if you take the 200 top 100m sprinters worldwide there is likely to be a large variation in BMI. However, if you take only the top ten there is likely to be very little variation. This indicates that through natural selection we are likely to be seeing optimum BMIs being developed for each running distance.

Recent modelling of BMI in male marathon runners also shows an inverse relationship between BMI and performance, around an optimal point. An increase or a decrease in BMI from an optimal point will lead to an decrement in performance.

Other anthropometrical factors that influence marathon-running performance are the ratio of leg length to sitting height, and the ratio between lower leg length and upper leg length. Essentially, marathon runners have long shins and calves with short thighs and upper bodies. This provides biomechanical efficiency. There is also evidence that a lower calf girth in runners leads to a decrease in running economy.

Interestingly, there is very little evidence to suggest that leanness determines exercise performance once below a certain threshold. So essentially, leaner is not always better, and there is likely to be an optimum for each individual.

There is therefore a clear link between body shape and size and running performance, and this is likely to be true for other sports and events. Of course, for sports where a weight category is important there is a clear need to manage body weight to comply with the rules of the sport. However, there is very little research in many sports to guide athletes on 'competition weight'.

131

WEIGHT MANAGEMENT

Although we may know or even accept that there is an optimum 'competition weight' for each athlete, it's the process of obtaining this weight that's the tricky part. Get this wrong and there are consequences for the body that will inhibit performance. The next section will look at the evidence base for weight loss in athletes.

How to lose weight

Weight loss is theoretically simple and follows the first law of thermodynamics, which states that energy cannot be created or destroyed. Therefore, when a human being is in energy balance, energy intake will match energy expenditure. It makes sense beyond this to assume that if you increase energy intake, while maintaining energy expenditure, weight gain will ensue. On the flip side, if you decrease energy intake and maintain energy expenditure, weight loss is inevitable.

Using this first law of thermodynamics, we can start to make some predictions on the size of weight loss and weight gain. First of all, let's look at weight gain. Let's take your average 70kg male with an energy expenditure of 2,500 kcal (this is the predicted average for your average Joe). If our average Joe increases his energy intake by only 10 kcal per day, this could be an over-consumption of food of 3,650 kcal per year. Let's take this assumption one step further and assume that all of this excess energy is stored as body fat. Body fat provides around 9 kcal per g of fat. Therefore, in theory, with this excess intake of only 10 kcal per day our average Joe will increase his body weight by 0.4kg. Increase this excess energy intake to 100 kcal per day, about the energy found in one small banana, then the weight increase would theoretically be 4kg; increase this to one muffin from your favourite coffee shop and that weight increase per year jumps to a whopping 18.5kg.

Let's flip this on its head now and assume these numbers are a calorie deficit per day. In theory, if you remove that muffin you have with your morning coffee you should lose 18.5kg per year. Simple. It's that easy.

I hope something in your mind right now is feeling a bit conflicted. When you break it down like this, weight gain and weight loss seem simple. Yet we all know that this is not the case.

The first law of thermodynamics is a law of nature and cannot be broken. Therefore, what is going on? If the problem is not necessarily the law itself, there must be something wrong with our measurements.

This is where things start to get a little bit murky and grey. First of all, there are real challenges in accurately gauging how much energy we consume each day in the food we eat. We can look at what we ate yesterday, but let's be honest, how much can you really remember? A food diary? This depends on the person recording it being accurate and not missing off that cheeky latte they had while out with their friends – not to mention the interpretation of portion sizes by the nutritionist doing the analysis. What if we took a diary for a few days and averaged it? Well, the day-to-day variation in total calorie intake in a human being is around 25 per cent, so averaging a diary might exclude some vital information. We could take photos of everything, which makes interpretation easier. Or we could weigh everything we eat. But who really wants to do that? So to start with, measuring energy intake is messy and fraught with potential error.

Let's make an assumption that we have got an accurate representation of food intake from an athlete. We then make calculations of calorie content of the food we consume from pre-determined norms. However, these norms have a natural variation about

WEIGHT MANAGEMENT

them as they are an average. Not only this, the energy that is received by the body for it to use is highly variable and dependent on many factors, including how much the food is cooked, how the food was grown, not to mention how much is absorbed as it passes through the stomach and intestine. As you can see, there is significant disconnect between the food we theoretically eat and the food we do consume.

What about energy expenditure? Surely this is easier to measure? Well, not really. Day-to-day energy expenditure varies by around about 8 per cent, so for our average Joe this would be a variation of 136 kcal per day. Energy expenditure is made up of three components:

- Basal metabolic rate: This is the energy we need just to survive if we don't do any exercise. This varies on average by 3.3 per cent per day. So taking our 70kg average Joe, this means on a daily basis the BMR could be plus or minus 56 kcal. BMR also decreases with age.

- Thermic effect of food: This is the amount of energy needed to digest and process the food we eat. It accounts for around 10 per cent of our energy expenditure, although this value is very variable depending on what type of food is consumed. For instance, if you consume carbohydrates or fat, 5–15 per cent of the energy consumed is used for digestion, but for protein it is 20–35 per cent. How processed the food is when consumed will also lead to a different thermic effect.

- Physical activity: This provides a significant amount of energy towards our daily energy needs. It is dependent on the type of exercise, fitness of the individual, body weight, intensity and duration of exercise.

We can see, therefore, that on both sides of the energy in and energy out equation there are challenges on the accurate measurement of both energy intake and expenditure. While the first law of thermodynamics definitely holds true, in practice it is very

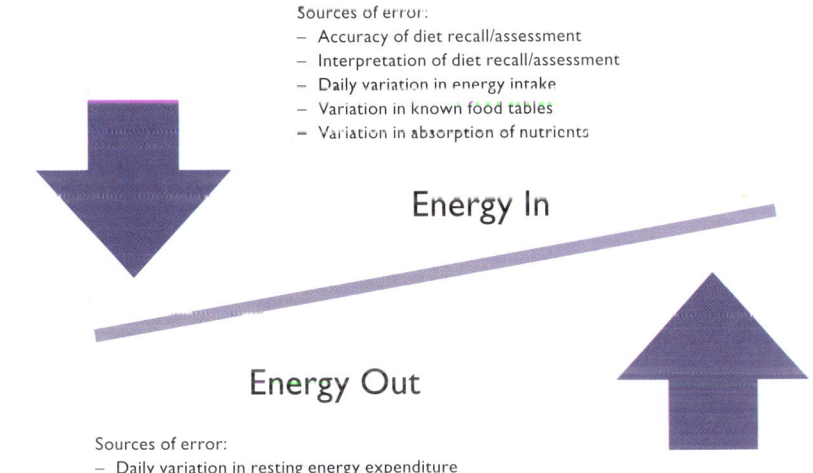

Sources of error:
- Accuracy of diet recall/assessment
- Interpretation of diet recall/assessment
- Daily variation in energy intake
- Variation in known food tables
- Variation in absorption of nutrients

Energy In

Energy Out

Sources of error:
- Daily variation in resting energy expenditure
- Thermic effect of food dependent on type of food eaten
- Physical activity and economy of movement

Sources of variation in energy expenditure and intake.

WEIGHT MANAGEMENT

hard to implement on a daily basis and ensure we will get weight loss or gain. Another factor also at play in the human body is the hormonal control of body composition and food intake. We will explore this area next.

Hormones and weight loss

Calories in and calories out makes theoretical sense. However, as we have seen, it is actually quite complicated. Now we are about to add another layer of complexity to the mix: hormones, those pesky signalling molecules that help us to regulate our bodies. As you can guess, they play a key role in regulating body composition and appetite. How they do this is even more complicated than calories in, calories out.

The stomach and intestine is the largest endocrine organ in the body. This means it produces a lot of hormones. In fact, the stomach and intestine is second only to our brain in terms of the number of neurons that are present. It has even been called our second brain.

When we eat food a whole series of hormones is released by the body to signal that food is on the way and we should control our eating. These have wonderful scientific acronyms such as CCK, PYY and GLP-1, to name just three. All three of these are actually part of the appetite regulation system of the body and are stimulated in response to food intake. Once stimulated they interact with the hypothalamus in particular to signal to us that we are full.

To make things a touch more complicated, what we eat leads to different responses from these appetite hormones. Protein leads to a larger increase in these hormones than does fat, which in turn leads to a greater stimulation than carbohydrate. The outcome is that protein makes you feel fuller and for longer, whereas carbohydrate is the least satiating nutrient.

In addition, there are signals that tell the body that we are hungry, in particular the hormone ghrelin – never mind signals from

---

RESEARCH FOCUS

Processed food and energy expenditure
Barr and Wright (2010) investigated the effects of how a food is processed prior to eating it on the increase in post-prandial energy expenditure – so in essence, how much energy it takes to digest the food in question. In this case the participants consumed two different cheese sandwiches on separate days. Both of these sandwiches contained 600 kcal and roughly the same proportions of carbohydrate, fat and protein. However, one of the sandwiches was made with wholegrain bread and cheddar cheese, the second with white bread and a processed cheese slice filling.

Both of the sandwiches reduced hunger and increased feelings of satiety to the same extent, but the wholefood sandwich was deemed more palatable than the processed meal of white bread and cheese. Post-meal ingestion energy expenditure increased significantly more, and by a longer period, when the wholefood meal was ingested. Of the energy consumed as part of the wholefood meal, 19.9 per cent of the energy consumed in the meal was converted to energy in the process of digestion, whereas only 10.7 per cent of the energy consumed in the white bread sandwich was burnt in digestion. The wholefood meal also kept the metabolic rate above baseline for an hour longer than the processed meal.

adipose tissue (fat stores, if you're not a scientist), such as leptin, which is generally released from adipose tissue to reduce hunger.

Insulin

Once this complex process of regulating appetite is in place, hormones begin to decide where and how the food we eat is stored. In particular the hormone insulin has a significant effect on the storage and use of food we consume. Put simply, insulin is our storage hormone. It is released from the pancreas in response to carbohydrate intake in particular, although can be stimulated by protein intake, too. It has a significant effect on metabolism throughout the body, including the muscle.

An increase in insulin will lead to storage of carbohydrate within the muscle in the form of muscle glycogen. Insulin is produced by the body, at least in a healthy state, in direct response to an increase in blood glucose, so that the body can regulate blood glucose concentrations. This is important as consistently high blood glucose can be toxic for the body.

Insulin also causes storage of glucose in adipose tissue. This is where some of the challenges start to come in. Not only will this ultimately lead to an increase in body fat, but increases in insulin inhibit the body's use of fat as a fuel. So in essence, excessive increases in insulin will cause storage of excess energy as fat and inhibit breakdown of fat.

From here we can start to see that control of insulin becomes important in our management of body weight. Excessively high insulin on a consistent basis will lead to an increase in body fat, but if we manage insulin appropriately we can start to control body weight. Next, we will look at how we can do this.

Insulin is released by the pancreas in response to an increase in blood sugar, primarily after the ingestion of carbohydrates (although it should be noted that proteins also elicit the release of insulin into the circulation). Different carbohydrates elicit a different insulin response after they have been eaten.

Let's take the simplest of carbohydrates, glucose. This is a simple sugar which when consumed rapidly appears in the bloodstream, leading to a rapid increase in blood sugar. This increase in blood sugar is detected in the pancreas and insulin is released into the bloodstream from the pancreas to reduce blood sugar back down to baseline levels.

However, when insulin appears in the blood there are a whole raft of physiological consequences, mainly aimed at speeding up the removal of sugar from the blood. Some of these are positive for athletes in that there will be an increase in muscle glycogen synthesis, therefore increasing the size of the fuel tank in the muscle. There will also be an increase in amino acid intake into the muscle, and an increase in blood flow around the body. All positive responses for an athlete.

However, there are other consequences that may not be as positive, especially if weight loss is the aim of the athlete. There will be an increase in fat storage within adipose tissue in the body; adipose tissue is the main storage space for fat and is the tissue you are trying to decrease in size when it comes to weight loss. Less fat will also be burnt as a fuel, and carbohydrate metabolism increased.

So due to this increase in insulin we have decreased our ability to burn fat, and increased storage of both carbohydrate and fat in adipose tissue. We have just made it harder for our bodies to get rid of the adipose tissue we are trying to dispose of in weight loss. If we do this as a one-off, say by drinking a can of Coca-Cola, there is likely to be very

WEIGHT MANAGEMENT

little long-term effect. The challenge comes when insulin spikes on a consistent basis, or just stays elevated because of the food we are eating.

The amount of insulin released depends on how much carbohydrate is consumed and what type. The example of glucose is one extreme, as it is the simplest of carbohydrates. If we take the other extreme and look at a carbohydrate which is absorbed relatively slowly, such as a lentil, then the increase in blood sugar in response to ingesting the lentil will be less. This will still lead to an increase in insulin, but to far less an extent.

The concept of speed of absorption of carbohydrates is generally termed the glycaemic index. The glycaemic index was first introduced by David Jenkins and his fellow researchers from the University of Toronto in 1981. It tracks the response of blood sugar in response to 50g of carbohydrate from a given food, and gives it a ranking compared to a reference food, which is normally 50g of glucose. A high glycaemic index is generally one which has a score of 70 or more; 56–69 are categorized as moderate, and less than 56 as low. So one simple way to control insulin is to make food choices that reduce the glycaemic index of carbohydrates.

Maintaining muscle mass during weight loss

Let's recap so far in terms of weight loss. We know we need to keep an energy deficit, even if this is hard to quantify. We need to make sure we don't get big troughs and peaks in our blood sugar, so keeping an eye on our carbohydrate intake is key. The next challenge we face is what type of body weight do we want to lose? In most athletic cases, the need is to lose body fat and retain as much muscle as we possibly can.

In general when you try and lose weight by cutting calories the body does not discriminate between fat and muscle in what it will lose. The greater the calorie deficit and therefore the greater the weight loss, the greater the percentage of the weight loss is muscle mass.

Another challenge for athletes is that it seems they are more susceptible to losing muscle mass during weight loss. This phenomenon is likely to be related to their starting body fat percentage. The leaner an athlete is when weight loss begins, the more that weight loss is likely to come from muscle mass rather than fat mass.

Muscle mass is regulated by the interaction of muscle protein synthesis (MPS) and muscle protein breakdown (MPB). When MPS is increased without an increase in MPB, muscle mass is gained. In the reverse situation where MPB is greater than MPS, muscle mass is lost. During periods of energy restriction nothing seems to happen to MPB. However, MPS is reduced.

Reduction in MPS during energy restriction occurs early in the restriction period and seems to continue to reduce until a plateau occurs. Building new muscle fibres is an energy-demanding process, so therefore it makes sense that in a period where energy may be scarce the body works to reduce MPS. During this early reduction of MPS in response to energy restriction, MPS is also less responsive to the protein we consume.

One way in which this decrease in MPS can be combatted is to increase protein intake at the weight-loss period. At least doubling the RDA (which stands at 0.9g/kg of body weight per day) appears to maintain MPS during energy restriction. While tripling the dose of protein to approximately 3g/kg of body weight per day does not provide additional benefits in healthy adults, it should not be ruled out

WEIGHT MANAGEMENT

for athletes. It is likely that an increase in protein intake will be necessary above an individual's baseline intake in order to maintain MPS, and as athletes will often have protein intakes that are higher than normal adults, it is likely that they will need this higher intake. Resistance exercise also appears to be beneficial in maintain MPS during energy restriction.

A fascinating study from the research group of Professor Kevin Tipton, then at the University of Birmingham, and conducted by Samuel Mettler, highlights this effect. Taking a group of resistance-trained athletes, they put them on a diet that caused a 40 per cent reduction in energy intake. One diet regime had protein intake of 2.3g/kg of body weight per day, the other had only 1g/kg of body weight per day. Those who ate the diet that was higher in protein maintained their muscle mass, and primarily lost fat weight. Those who had a lower intake of protein also lost similar amounts of muscle mass.

As we saw in Chapter 3 when investigating the desire to increase muscle mass, the individual amount and distribution of protein intake is key. As overall protein intake needs to be increased, either the amount or frequency of protein intake needs to be increased too. Assuming an athlete is already consuming five or six meals and snacks with approximately 20–30g of protein in them, it is clear that the amount of protein will need to be increased. Aim for an intake of approximately 0.4g/kg of body weight per serving.

What if weight loss goes wrong?

There are times when an athlete has to make a certain weight, no matter what. This is particularly the case in weight-managed sports such as combat sports or lightweight rowing. While it is perfectly possible to lose weight and maintain performance to hit these targets, there are some potential pitfalls that should be considered.

Short-term strategies

Short-term strategies to lose body weight are common in weight-managed sports. Primarily, these revolve around extreme fluid and food restriction for one or two days prior to competition. They can take a variety of forms, which all involve trying to reduce body weight rapidly by reducing the body's water levels and muscle glycogen stores. These can include exercising in many layers of clothes or plastic bags, sitting in saunas to increase fluid loss, as well as just reducing food and fluid intake.

These practices have many physiological and psychological effects, which could be seen as being detrimental to performance. It is reported that short-term memory, concentration and vigour all decrease, along with increases in confusion and fatigue – not adaptations, which are preferable for athletic performance.

However, some psychological advantages could be conferred by certain weight-loss strategies. A study published in the *Journal of Athletic Training* in 2013 from scientists at the University of Gothenburg in Sweden explored the reasoning behind weight-loss strategies in fourteen elite Swedish combat sport athletes. Semi-structured interviews by the authors revealed that the athletes see these practices as part of their identity and that they provide a mental advantage over their competitors. Clearly, it is not as simple as saying that extreme weight-loss practices are negative, and thought must be put into any changes that may be made.

Physiological adaptations also occur where there is a decrease in plasma volume, a reduction in muscle glycogen concentration and hormonal and electrolyte imbalances. All of

WEIGHT MANAGEMENT

these have been shown to decrease both aerobic and anaerobic performance. However, their effect on the explosive performances needed in many combat sports is unclear. This is especially so as, with effective post-weigh-in nutrition practices, many of these physiological functions can be restored. This does depend on the schedule of the competition, though, which will dictate both the frequency of weigh-in and the time between weigh-in and competition.

Adaptation to rapid weight loss

There is some potential in the theory that athletes become habituated to continually undergoing rapid weight loss. Some evidence in the literature shows that those who are used to undertaking rapid weight-loss techniques can perform perfectly well despite the weight loss. It is possible that while the physiological changes to rapid weight loss continue, the perceptual responses reduce and therefore the athlete is still able to perform. This is especially so as restoring the physiological effects of rapid weight loss is relatively simple.

Chronic weight loss

Long-term calorie deficits can have devastating effects on the physiological functions of the body, as we saw in Chapter 2 in the context of the female athlete. In 2014 the International Olympic Committee Medical Commission issued a position stand highlighting the dangers of relative energy deficiency in sport and the potential negative consequences this could have on a range of performance and physiological factors.

One of the main challenges of undergoing a long-term energy deficit to achieve weight loss is that it is not only fat mass which is decreased but lean mass too. Lean mass is important for many aspects of sporting performance and therefore it is important to maintain as much as possible throughout a period of weight loss. As mentioned earlier, adequate protein intake will be vital to support this.

RAPID WEIGHT LOSS, RECOVERY AND LIGHTWEIGHT ROWING PERFORMANCE

Of interest is a series of studies from Dr Gary Slater of the Australian Institute of Sport investigating the effects of rapid weight-loss techniques on rowing performance. The first in the series of studies showed that acutely reducing body weight by 4 per cent reduced 2,000m rowing performance but only slightly, though the effects were greater in the heat. Interestingly, when a 2,000m time trial was performed on water, rather than on an ergometer, there was virtually no decrement in performance when reducing body weight then aggressively replenishing food and fluid.

In a follow-up study lightweight rowers were asked to reduce their body weight by 5.2 per cent prior to three separate weigh-ins and time trials. After weigh-in, the rowers were given either 2.2g per kg of carbohydrate, 28.5ml of fluid per kg of body weight or a combination of both. When fluid and carbohydrate were combined, and when only fluid was given, there was no decrement in performance compared to the pre-weigh-in time trial. However, carbohydrate only showed a decrement in performance. This seems to show that fluid replacement may be more important than carbohydrate replacement post-weight loss. However, both together also seem to be effective.

WEIGHT MANAGEMENT

Ina Garthe and colleagues of the Norwegian School of Sport Sciences in Oslo investigated the effects of two speeds of weight loss on body composition changes, along with strength and power measures. Twenty-four athletes undertook one of two different weight-loss protocols. One led to a weekly weight loss of 0.7 per cent of body mass, and a second 1.4 per cent of body mass. To achieve this, energy intake was decreased by 19 per cent in the slow weight-loss group and 30 per cent in the fast weight-loss group.

In both groups weight loss was around 5.5 per cent. In both changes in lean mass and fat mass, the slow rate of weight loss was more effective when compared to the fast group. When weight loss was at a rate of 0.7 per cent, fat mass decreased by 31 per cent compared to 21 per cent in the faster group. Lean mass also increased in the slow group by 2.1 per cent and did not change at all in the fast group. Across a number of different markers of performance, losing weight at the slower rate led to significant improvements in performance, such as a 7 per cent increase in counter-movement jumps compared to no change in the fast group.

This suggests that to maintain and even improve performance, attempting to lose weight at a rate of approximately 0.7 per cent of body weight per week is optimal. Interestingly, the slow weight loss group on average had a calorie deficit of 469 kcal per day. This is close to the general recommendations for weight loss of 500 kcal per day.

Weight maintenance

Once a desired body weight has been obtained, it should be maintained. How is this achieved? Simply, by eating as is appropriate for the training. There is no need to go crazy, no need to do anything radical. The aim should always be to eat appropriately for your training and competition needs. So go back to the aim of what you are trying to do and eat in the appropriate manner.

Other approaches

You know you want that six-pack, but it is just not working out for you. Time and time again you've tried the latest fad, you've gone Paleo, fasted intermittently, Venice Beach is done, and you've even lived off broccoli soup or whatever the latest craze is.

You pick up your latest sporting magazine. Any will do – could be a running, cycling or football magazine – it doesn't really matter. As you flick through the pages an advert stands out. Take this pill and magically you will have a six-pack, probably in five minutes. Have you seen these adverts?

Let's take a look at the evidence behind 'fat burning' supplements.

Well, that was a long paragraph, I was concerned it might eat into this book's word limit. I even considered not mentioning fat burning supplements whatsoever, so lacking in any scientific evidence are they, particularly when it comes to long-term sustainable weight loss. Don't be conned into buying them. The best way to increase the amount of fat you burn on a daily basis is exercise and this magic bullet called food.

Summary

- Body weight is made up of many components, and is highly variable both from day to day and within a day. At times body weight may change but little change in fat and muscle mass occurs, misleading the athlete.

139

WEIGHT MANAGEMENT

- Different performances need different body shapes for optimal performance and there is considerable individual variation in what is needed. There is a link between body shape and performance. However, it is not a simple relationship.
- Weight loss is theoretically simple and involves consuming fewer calories than are expended during day-to-day living. However, measuring the amount of calories consumed and expended is fraught with pitfalls and errors. At times this equation can therefore seem invalid.
- Weight loss is also complicated by the hormonal response to different foods. Appetite hormones are released by the gut in response to different foods.
- Insulin can play a role in weight management. Insulin acts as our storage hormone, and large increases in insulin can lead to storage of excess body fat.
- Weight loss can be a risk for athletes. Both short-term and long-term strategies for weight loss have their pros and cons. Care should be taken when embarking on a weight-loss regimen.
- There is no evidence for the use of 'fat burning' supplements to help lose weight.

Gold

Calorie deficit: The most important component of weight loss is to achieve a negative calorie balance. There is no magic bullet. Aim for a deficit of 500–1,000 kcal per day for optimum weight loss. Larger deficits may lead to a loss of muscle mass and performance. Physiological function may also be compromised.

Protein for weight loss: Protein is potentially the most important nutrient to promote weight loss. Increases in protein in the diet to 3g per kg of body weight per day will help to maintain muscle during weight loss. This

Meal	Food
Breakfast	3-egg omelette with ham 1 black coffee 1 priobiotic yogurt
Post-Exercise	20g of whey protein with 35g of carbohydrates
Lunch	1 baked salmon with a large salad
Snack	2 slices of wholemeal bread with almond butter
Post-Exercise	1 pint of semi-skimmed milk made into a smoothie with blueberries
Dinner	1 chicken breast with broccoli, kale and carrots
Pre-bed snack	125g pot of Greek yogurt

Carbohydrate (g/kg body weight) 1.9	Protein (g/kg body weight) 2.5	Fat (g/kg body weight) 1.2

WEIGHT MANAGEMENT

protein intake will also promote positive changes in appetite hormones, which will make the plan more satiating.

Low GI foods for weight loss: Decreasing the glycaemic index of carbohydrates will also promote weight loss through promoting satiety and regulating hormones such as insulin.

Further reading

Josse, A. R., Atkinson, S. A., Tarnopolsky, M. A. & Phillips, S. M. (2012). Diets higher in dairy foods and dietary protein support bone health during diet- and exercise-induced weight loss in overweight and obese premenopausal women. *The Journal of Clinical Endocrinology and Metabolism*, 97(1), 251–60. doi:10.1210/jc.2011-2165

Mettler, S., Mitchell, N. & Tipton, K. D. (2010). Increased Protein Intake Reduces Lean Body Mass Loss during Weight Loss in Athletes. *Medicine & Science in Sports & Exercise*, (326), 326–337. doi:10.1249/MSS.0b013e3181b2ef8e

Mountjoy, M., Sundgot-Borgen, J., Burke, L., Carter, S., Constantini, N., Lebrun, C., Ljungqvist, A. (2014). The IOC consensus statement: beyond the Female Athlete Triad–Relative Energy Deficiency in Sport (RED-S). *British Journal of Sports Medicine*, 48(7), 491–7. doi:10.1136/bjsports-2014-093502

Sedeaud, A., Marc, A., Marck, A., Dor, F., Schipman, J., Dorsey, M., Toussaint, J.-F. (2014). BMI, a performance parameter for speed improvement. *PloS One*, 9(2), e90183. doi:10.1371/journal.pone.0090183

INDEX

antioxidants 18–19, 65–66, 73, 80–81, 115, 123, 127
Beta-Alanine 38, 56, 108–110
caffeine 28, 39, 52, 54–55, 65, 79–80, 99–100, 102
carbohydrate 34, 43, 57, 118–120
   altitude 102–103
   brain 77–79, 83
   creatine 34–35
   during exercise 95–99
   heat 101–102
   immunity 15–18, 20
   injury 29
   interval training 53–54, 55–56
   mouth swilling 64–65
   pre exercise 90–93
   protein synthesis 45–46
   recovery 111–113, 121
   sleep 123–124
   training adaptations 51–52
   weight loss 134–136
colostrum 13–15, 20, 71, 95
creatine 30, 34–37, 54, 81
energy 10–11, 27, 31, 134,
   availability 11, 22–25
   deprivation 10
   and muscle mass 40
   and weight loss 132–134, 136, 138–39
fat 19, 40, 53–54, 65, 87, 135–137
   caffeine 99
   omega 3 29, 30
FODMAP 15, 38
Gastrointestinal distress 93–95
glutamine 15, 20, 71, 95
HMB 30, 38
hydration 70, 82, 88–90, 93, 101, 125
iron 68–69, 70–71
nitrates 26, 29, 73, 100–101
phosphataditic acid 39
probiotics 12–-3, 14, 20, 71
protein 25–26
   bone 28–29
   concurrent training 51–52
   fasted training 64–65
   hypertrophy 40–46
   muscle mass maintenance 30, 136–137
   post exercise 66–68
   recovery 113–115
sodium bicarbonate 56, 110–111
tyrosine 81
vitamins 18–19, 72–73, 83, 101, 116
   vitamin D 28

RELATED TITLES FROM CROWOOD

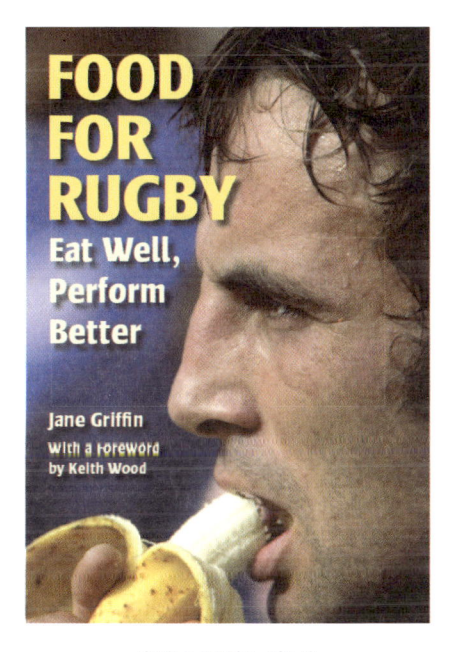

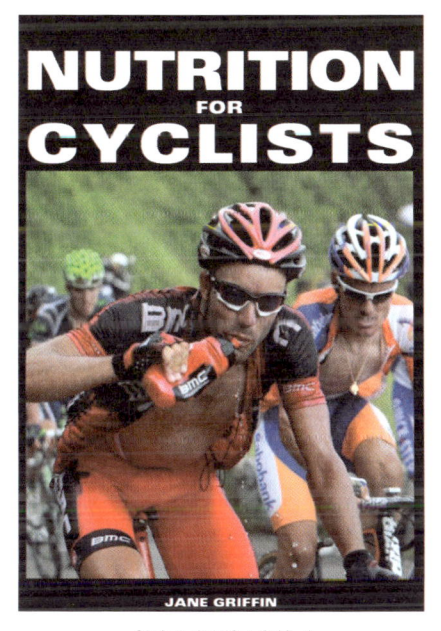

FOOD FOR RUGBY
Eat Well, Perform Better
Jane Griffin
With a Foreword by Keith Wood

978 1 86126 695 8

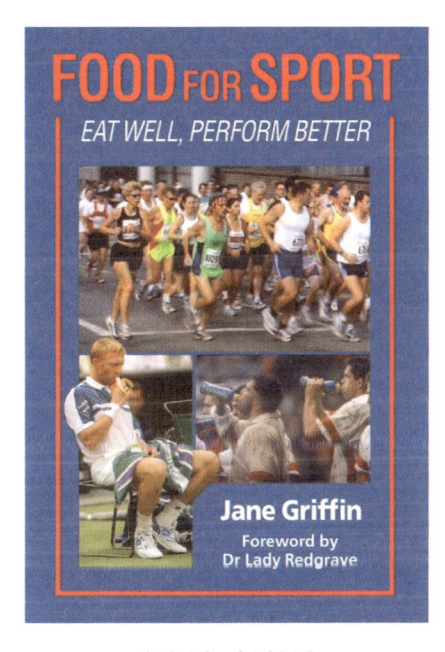

FOOD FOR SPORT
EAT WELL, PERFORM BETTER
Jane Griffin
Foreword by Dr Lady Redgrave

978 1 86126 216 5

NUTRITION FOR CYCLISTS
JANE GRIFFIN

978 1 84797 842 4

NUTRITION FOR MARATHON RUNNING
JANE GRIFFIN

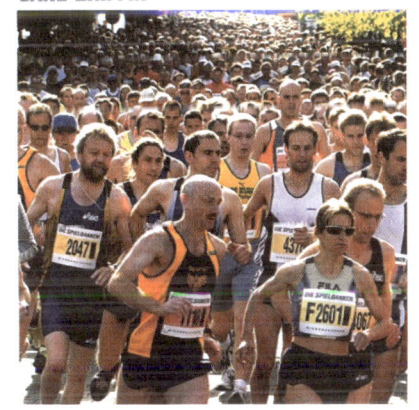

978 1 86126 590 6